"Anger is one of the biggest issues for relationships. *This book is must reading* ... *issues as well as for any professional interested in the prevention and treatment of relationship issues."*

Howard J. Markman, Ph.D.
Codirector, Center for Marital and Family Studies
University of Denver
Co-author, *Fighting* for *Your Marriage*

"A 'must-use book' for those who are serious about managing their anger more effectively. Chock full of practical suggestions and tools. I look forward to guiding my patients to this book. A great job!"

Robert J. Hedaya, M.D.
Clinical Professor of Psychiatry, Georgetown University
Hospital, Washington, D.C. Founder, National Center
for Whole Psychiatry,
Chevy Chase, Maryland
Author of *The Anti-Depressant Survival Program* and
Understanding Biological Psychiatry

"An excellent book. Dr. Schiraldi breaks new ground in exploring the different dimensions of anger and its management. I know of no other book that covers it with such clarity and detail. I will highly recommend it to all my patients."

Carlos Sandoval, M.D.
Director, Psychosocial Oncology Services
Silvestro Comprehensive Cancer Center
University of Miami

"A very useful compilation of practical techniques for emotional self-control. Highly recommended for personal and group use in any format where establishing more conscious control of mood states is a desired outcome."

Al Bacchus, Ph.D.
Program Coordinator, Corporate Health and Wellness Training
Montgomery College, Rockville, Maryland

The
Anger
Management
Sourcebook

GLENN R. SCHIRALDI, PH.D.
AND MELISSA HALLMARK KERR, PH.D.

Contemporary Books

Chicago   New York   San Francisco   Lisbon   London   Madrid   Mexico City
Milan   New Delhi   San Juan   Seoul   Singapore   Sydney   Toronto

Library of Congress Cataloging-in-Publication Data

Schiraldi, Glenn R., 1947-
    The anger management sourcebook / Glenn R. Schiraldi & Melissa
Hallmark Kerr.
        p.   cm.
    Includes bibliographical references and index.
    ISBN 0-7373-0591-6
    1. Anger. I. Kerr, Melissa Hallmark. II. Title.

    BF575.A5 S35   2002
    152.4'7—dc21   2002020115

Contemporary Books

A Division of The McGraw·Hill Companies

6 7 8 9 0 DOC/DOC 1 0 9 8 7 6 5 4

ISBN 0-7373-0591-6

This book was set in Sabon by Rattray Design
Printed and bound by R. R. Donnelley—Crawfordsville

Cover design by Jeanette Wojtyla

McGraw-Hill books are available at special quantity discounts to use as premiums and
sales promotions, or for use in corporate training programs. For more information, please
write to the Director of Special Sales, Professional Publishing, McGraw-Hill, Two Penn
Plaza, New York, NY 10121-2298. Or contact your local bookstore.

This book is intended to provide accurate and authoritative information and teach skills that
will benefit a wide range of people. However, it is not a substitute for competent professional
help, when such help is needed. We suggest that readers consult a qualified and experienced mental health professional for spousal or child abuse or other forms of violence; for
clinical depression, anxiety, or other forms of mental illness; or for continuing relationship difficulties that do not resolve despite their best efforts.

Contents

Acknowledgments

IT IS A JOY to have the opportunity to write a book such as this, to combine our experience and the experience of so many gifted researchers and practitioners in producing a resource that we hope will be of use to others.

We first thank those participants at the Pentagon and the University of Maryland who patiently helped us wrestle with turning the theory of anger management into practice and refine the methods of teaching anger management.

We are thankful to Drs. Aaron T. Beck and Albert Ellis for their pioneering work in detailing the relationship between our thoughts and afflictive emotions. We are also thankful to famous people such as Mother Teresa, the Dalai Lama, Martin Luther King, Jr., Arthur Ashe, Mohandas Gandhi, and Albert Schweitzer—as well as every-day people, parents, friends, workers, drivers—who lived or are living the beautiful opposites of problem anger. They wittingly or unwittingly were and are teachers of patience and compassion.

We are extremely grateful to those who have generously given of their time to review this book and provide helpful suggestions: Drs. Al Bacchus, Robert J. Hedaya, Bruce B. Hill, Howard Markman, Tinsley W. Rucker, Carlos Sandoval, and Mohammad Beiraghdar. And Denis M. Ceritos, Carina Deans, Clara Martin, Careen R. Mayer, and

Grace Zemba. And finally, thanks to Hudson Perigo, Rena Copperman, and all the staff at Contemporary/McGraw-Hill for your encouragement and meticulous attention to detail.

Portions of this book are adapted from Dr. Schiraldi's previous works, and first person references to an author throughout the book refer to Dr. Schiraldi unless otherwise noted.

Introduction

ROAD RAGE . . . computer rage . . . couples conflict and domestic violence . . . blowups with coworkers, supervisors, and children . . . bullying . . . school violence . . . child abuse . . . lack of civility . . . rampant litigation . . . terrorism and other hate crimes. This might indeed be called the Age of Problem Anger.

Problem anger is the Great Destroyer. A seemingly uncontrollable fire, it destroys relationships, careers, health, and inner peace. It saps the joy of living, leaves one feeling ashamed and foolish, and turns everyday challenges into explosive battlegrounds. These negative consequences of problem anger need not occur.

Why is there so much anger? Why do I get so angry? How can I break the vicious cycles of anger and get off the anger treadmill?

The good news is that much has been learned about anger in recent years. We now understand both its causes and the ways to reduce it. If anger is causing problems in your life, it is not because you are defective or a bad person. You simply may have not yet mastered the critical skills needed to manage this complex emotion.

This book will help you make your journey through life more calm, peaceful, and rich. With less anger, you will be more level-headed, making better decisions and maintaining more self-control. You will guard your health by reducing the risks of cardiovascular disease and other stress-related medical illnesses.[1] Most importantly, you will enjoy life more and have better relationships with others.

You will become skilled at recognizing your choice to become angry or not, at choosing effective alternatives to anger, and at constructively channeling the energy of anger into productive thoughts, feelings, and behaviors. You will learn how to become angry for the right purpose, with the right person, at the right time, to the right degree, and in the right way. You will develop greater inner peace so as to be less prone to becoming angry—able to function more calmly, without overreacting.

Because anger is a universal emotion, this book is of special interest to all who wish to lessen the destructive effects of excessive anger. It will be especially useful to people who become angry in traffic, at work, at home, or at play, and who wish to be more effective in these situations. Regulation of your feelings, especially anger, will help you become a more effective parent, spouse, friend, teacher, leader, and coworker. If you are at risk for high blood pressure, heart disease, or other anger-related illnesses, this book may indeed be lifesaving. It will be especially useful if your profession frequently exposes you to provocative situations, such as police work or the military, and to the many members of support groups, ranging from incest survivors to parents of murdered children.

This book will also be an invaluable resource to health professionals who counsel those with problem anger, including physicians, physicians' assistants, psychologists, psychiatrists, social workers, marriage and family therapists, pastoral counselors, mental health counselors, occupational therapists, expressive art therapists, critical incident debriefing specialists, health educators, and graduate students preparing for these professions.

PART I

Understanding Anger

1

About Anger

There is nobody who lives happily with anger.

—Shantideva

What Is Anger?

Anger is a universal, natural, and understandable emotion. The dictionary describes anger as an unpleasant and uncomfortable feeling resulting from injury, mistreatment, or opposition and usually showing itself in a desire to fight back at the supposed cause of the feeling. Anger involves:

- *Thoughts* that trigger and/or maintain anger. Anger is likely to be greater if one presumes an offense to be wrong, deliberate, or preventable, creating great hardship and/or deserving punishment. The thought that one's anger is justified also tends to intensify anger.

- *Physiological arousal*, such as flushed face, increased heart rate and blood pressure, sweating, and the release of various stress hormones.

- *Behaviors* or tendencies to act that are culturally influenced, such as yelling, clenching fists, or pouting.

- *The apparent purpose of protecting or furthering our self-interests*, which might include loved ones, causes, or cherished principles.

Anger is a secondary emotion, meaning it is preceded by other feelings, such as pain or fear. A close look at the word reveals some of anger's subtleties. Anger has the same root as *anguish* (meaning agony and distress) and *angst* (meaning anxious fear), suggesting its unpleasant nature and origin. Think of an angry wound, and you'll probably get an image of one that is sensitive and painful. In fact, a second definition of anger is an inflammation of a sore or wound, suggesting the source of some forms of anger. Anger is called an afflictive emotion because it is associated with pain, suffering, injury, or distress. Anger derives from words that mean constricted, narrow, tightness, strangle, and squeeze. The fact that anger correlates with anxiety and depression further suggests that it can be a symptom of pain.

Anger can be characterized by its:

- *Frequency*. The average adult gets angry once a day, and annoyed about three times a day.

- *Intensity*. Anger can range from mild (agitated, annoyed, irritated) to strong (fury, rage).

- *Duration*. How long do you stay angry after you get angry? Do you cool down quickly or do you take a long time to recover? Do you hold grudges? Is your anger usually temporary or long lasting?

- *Threshold*. It takes a lot to get some people angry, while others react to fairly minimal provocations.

- *Expression*. Individuals vary in the way they manifest anger.
  - Some express anger in a rather muted, calm way.
  - Others boil inside but suffer in silence.
  - Some let people know of their anger in dramatic ways (e.g., scream, throw things, dilate their nostrils, give icy glares).
  - Some have an icy cold anger, without apparent outward expression.

- Some make snide comments, talk negatively about others, frequently complain about life's unfairness, become tense, or retaliate.

- *Degree of comfort.* Some dislike the feeling of anger, some are relatively comfortable with it, and some may even find aspects of anger empowering or invigorating.

Conditions Related to Anger

Aggression

Anger may or may not lead to aggression, or forceful behavior. Not all aggression is destructive or harmful. *Aggressive* means full of enterprise or initiative; bold, active, pursuing goals, self-confident. For example, one might aggressively insist on driving a drunken friend home. Here the intent is to help or protect, so the aggressive behavior is not considered hostile or destructive. We must look at the intent and the nature of the behavior to determine if aggression is destructive. Destructive, or hostile, aggression is associated with:

- Deliberate intent to harm, attack, injure, hurt, dominate, and/or control
- Actions that harm/hurt oneself or others (e.g., smashing one's own computer, violence, hitting, shoving, cutting, throwing things, using words to belittle or hurt)
- Starting fights or arguments
- Being ruthless, pushy, or militant
- Bullying. According to Fried and Fried, this is described by behavior:[1]

  - That intends to harm
  - That maintains power through size, age, strength, and/or gender
  - Where the victim is vulnerable, isolated, and/or exposed
  - Where the intensity and duration are such that the victim responds with damaged self-esteem, withdrawal, or aggression

- Dangerous driving (forcing drivers off the road, cutting others off, speeding)
- Teasing, or making threats or insults

Passive Aggression

This is angry behavior that is indirect and oftimes confusing. For various reasons, people might not choose to directly confront an offender. For example, they might feel they are lacking in power, or fear confrontation, so they might disguise their anger by:

- Using sarcasm, jokes, or teasing ("Oh, I was only fooling.")
- Spreading rumors
- Asking "innocent" questions ("Did you gain some weight?")
- Feigning confusion, tiredness, headache, concern ("You look tired.")
- Being late to intentionally annoy someone
- Forgetting or using other excuses ("I was caught in traffic.")
- Saying, "You're right" (when they don't mean it)
- "Accidentally" burning dinner, losing something that belongs to you, or wrecking your car
- Slamming drawers while saying that nothing is wrong

Hostility

Hostility is a relatively enduring attitude toward other people, resulting in the view that others are bad, immoral, untrustworthy, and selfish. It amounts to dislike, cynicism, suspicion, prejudice, and enmity. Hostility fuels anger by assuming that people will do bad things. One then prepares to react by withdrawing, defending, or mounting an offense. Hostility is often accompanied by ill will— the desire to hurt, get even, blame, wish ill fortune to another, or punish. Did you ever stop to think how you punish people with whom you are angry? Some complain, criticize, scold, give the cold shoulder, withhold affection, or cut off "bad" drivers. You can detect hostility by hearing words like, "She can screw herself"; "What a moron. I hope he gets arrested." Hostility has been linked to cardiovascular disease, and increased risk of death from many causes.

Summary

From the above it might be evident that anger takes many forms. It might occur with or without aggression; with or without hostility. For some, anger might be relatively situational—evident only in certain provoking situations. For others, anger might be generalized, so that they are chronically angry much or most of the time—prone to irritability, crankiness, and ill-temper; angry with many things; and complaining, critical, and argumentative. Some deny they are angry when they are. Some disown their anger or their role in it ("I'm not the problem. You are!"). Some displace their anger to other people or causes. And some are comfortable in acknowledging it and expressing it in appropriate ways.

What Triggers Anger?

Imagine that you are a trout swimming up a clear stream. In the water are many hooks from people who are fishing along the banks. Some of the hooks have lost their bait and hold little interest for you. Some have rather uninteresting bait. Others are colorful lures that are very inviting. You have several choices. You can swim right by the hooks and pay little attention. You can swim around other hooks curiously without biting. You can nibble at others. Or you can swallow the hooks whole and struggle mightily.

The hooks represent stressors, or triggers that "get you angry." Hooks fall under four categories. One might be angry at:

1. *Others*, when they hurt us or don't do what we expect of them.
2. *Situations*, such as traffic jams, getting lost, a computer glitch, losing something, frustrated goals, interruptions, or an injustice.

3. *Self.* One of the greatest fears is disappointing oneself for failing to meet personal goals. Anger ensues from not acknowledging our realistic limitations. To say "I can't believe I'm so stupid. Why can't I do that?" means "I won't accept my own fallibility."
4. *A combination of the above.* For example, frustration at a traffic jam might turn into anger at other drivers and then yourself for getting so angry.

It is interesting to ask: "Are you harder on yourself or on others regarding mistakes?" Most people say themselves, because they know their own potential. However, when asked about inconsiderate drivers, many people change their minds. Do you have a double standard? Or are you equally hard on yourself and others?

What are your hooks? Take a few moments to identify your greatest irritants. List these on a sheet of paper. Exhibit 1.1 lists hooks that have been identified by groups of adults over the years. As you consider your hooks, you might notice the following: First, your hooks are not new. People have gotten angry at similar situations many times in the past. It might help to realize that you are not unusual. Second, if you are like most people, you probably identified hooks that are external to yourself. You might have identified poor drivers as your hook. Rarely do we identify hooks as our own readiness to be angry, insecure, or self-doubting. Viewed this way, hooks can be great teachers to point out what we can strengthen in ourselves. Third, rate from 0 to10 how much power you have to control the nature of your hooks. A 10 means you have total control and 0 means you have none. For example, if you identified rude drivers and you made an all-out effort to control their poor driving, just how much could you actually control their poor driving? The truth is that we often have very little control over hooks, and almost never have total control. Simply realizing this and accepting that fact is somewhat calming. Ask, "Why should I make myself crazy over things I can't control?" The real power comes from controlling our inner lives.

The bottom line is, *Which is the greater threat—the hook or my reaction to it?* We might ask:

Exhibit 1.1 Hooks

Identifying the source of anger is an important step to managing anger. Anger triggers—whether they be others, situations, or self—threaten our needs or desires that we consider important. Notice what is threatened by these hooks: dignity, self-esteem, safety, intimacy, independence, comfort, rights, feeling in control/powerful/efficacious, stature/reputation, and/or sense of fairness.

"I get most angry at . . ."

Authority figures
Backstabbing
Being abandoned
Being cheated
Being ignored or slighted; getting the
    brush-off
Being kept waiting
Being lied to or misled
Being smothered, dominated, controlled
    by another
Being threatened, bullied, or intimidated
Being used, exploited, manipulated, taken
    advantage of (e.g., someone doesn't
    return a loan)
Being wronged; unfairness
Being wrongly blamed
Betrayal
Bossy bosses
Broken promises
Challenge to my authority, wisdom;
    someone dismisses my opinion
Change, uncertainty
Chaos, confusion, lack of order
Cherished belief challenged or disparaged
Complaining
Computer snafu/malfunction
Criticism, contempt, putdown, insult,
    belittled, devalued
Deadlines
Delays, being late, running late
Disapproval
Disobedient children
Disruptions

Favoritism
Feeling anxious, depressed, or guilty
Forced to do something against my will
Frustrated goals, don't get my way
Getting lost
Getting the silent treatment
God
Gossip
Humiliation, embarrassment, others know
    my weaknesses, made to look foolish
Imposition
Incompetence—mine or others
Inconsiderate behaviors (reckless or
    aggressive driving, vulgarity, profanity,
    playing music loudly, cutting in lines,
    selfishness)
Interference with meeting my goals (e.g.,
    fools who get in my way)
Interruptions
Jealousy
Lazy people who don't pull their weight
Letting myself down
Losing an argument
Losing athletic competition
Losing control
Losing something
Loss of love
Loud noise, noisy people, other
    distractions
Memories (irritating, painful, etc.)
Missed desired promotion
Nagging
Overload, pressure

Exhibit 1.1 (Continued)

Overwhelmed, over my head, out of control, powerlessness	Pushy, demanding, or aggressive people
People don't tell me what they're upset about	Rejection
	Reprimands
People in express lane at supermarket with too many items	Rude, discourteous, inconsiderate people
	Seeing others treated unjustly
	Slow drivers
People let me down, fall short of my standards, don't take responsibility	Spouse walks away when I try to talk to him/her
People who take out their anger on me	Traffic jams, bottlenecks
Performing below my capacity or expectations	Unclear expectations by boss
	Unsolicited advice
Personal ineptitude—especially when others can do it	Wasting time at meetings
	Weaknesses in others (indecision, dependence, dishonesty, etc.)
Prejudice, racism	

- Is it really such a big deal to not get what I assume I *must* have? Is this really critical to my basic survival? Can I like myself and live happily despite the world's flaws?

- Which is more important: To get my way or to live patiently in an imperfect world?

Why Does Anger Arise?

The causes of anger are understandable. They make sense. Understanding the root causes helps us to know which interventions will be needed. There are four primary causes of anger and nine secondary factors. Your anger likely arises from several of these acting in combination.

Primary Factors: The Core Four Causes

1. *We care.* People who become angry reflect a will to live, to grow, and to protect self-interests. Anger can also arise from a desire to protect other people or cherished causes or principles, such as jus-

tice. If we did not care, we would cease to react. Caring is a whole-some quality, a strength to maintain. As we will see, however, there are ways to channel that caring with less anger or no anger at all.

2. *Self-diminishment* underlies much problem anger. It can be very painful to feel rejected, disrespected, powerless, like a nobody; to be reminded of our own inadequacies or unworthiness. In the extreme, such feelings can trigger the fear of extinction. When angry, ask yourself, "How vulnerable do I now feel? What painful feeling lies beneath the anger?"

3. *Anger temporarily numbs the pain of self-diminishment.* Anger attempts to restore lost power. However, anger does not neu-tralize our feeling of inadequacy or powerlessness, at least not for long. It does not earn the deep love or respect we desire, or give us the power we want. Instead anger may increase our sense of pow-erlessness. For example, we give power to others to make us mad. Or, we scream at a computer, which of course does not respond.

4. *Unrealistic expectations.* Think about this one. How much of your anger arises from expecting too much? Do you expect other drivers to be more perfect than they are? Do you expect to have more control than you actually do? Do you expect yourself to be more perfect than you obviously are?

Entitlement is a special form of unrealistic expectations. Entitle-ment is the sense that the world owes us something without our hav-ing to work for it, and is reflected in thoughts such as "I shouldn't be hurt, corrected, or criticized"; "I should have advantages over others after all I've been through"; "I shouldn't have to work so hard."

Much anger, therefore, arises from a failure to accept the way things truly are. You, other people, and the world are and always will be imperfect. Accepting this fact reduces much anger.

Secondary Factors

Anger tends to be intensified by the existence of any of the follow-ing factors:

1. *Hot buttons* are unhealed emotional wounds or unresolved pain from the past. Perhaps someone has "pushed your button" and evoked a reaction that seemed disproportionate to the situation, and asked, "Where did all that anger come from?" Perhaps you carry low self-esteem, a sense of inadequacy, feelings of abandonment, unhappiness, or dissatisfaction with your life's course. Perhaps weaknesses in others remind you of similar weaknesses in yourself that have caused you pain in the past. For example, perhaps you were once criticized or felt ashamed for being indecisive, weak, nonassertive, depressed, or incompetent. When you see these traits in loved ones you become angry, hoping to put an end to them. Or the weakness of another person might remind you of your powerlessness to help. When you see pain in others you try to defend against your pain with anger. You might futilely try to change them with your anger. However, these buttons remain emotionally charged until we touch the wounds and pain in ourselves and others with compassion. Hot buttons remind us that anger is a secondary emotion. Underneath the anger is fear and/or pain.

2. *Family or personal history.* Children tend to repeat behaviors that they have seen modeled. Perhaps in the family you grew up in adults or siblings frequently flew off the handle, and you learned their habits. Perhaps you saw people rewarded for their anger, such as an Army officer who caused people to jump when he became angry (so you learned that anger seems to get you what you want). In your family, you might have experienced neglect, abandonment, or poor attachment, causing pain and eventually anger to arise.

3. *Preconceived cognitions* are certain thinking habits that intensify anger. If one tends to think of offenses as deliberate, mean-spirited, personal, and inexcusable then anger is more likely to be extreme. When people have the habit of hostility they are more likely to take offense because they already distrust other persons' motives. Many people rationalize anger ("She's a feisty redhead—it's cute"; "It's our family's way—no one messes with me"; "Anger is the only way to get her off my back").

4. *Excessive self-focus* can take several forms. One may think, "I want things *my* way, on *my* time." Such people seem indifferent to the needs of others. Some people create an inflated sense of self (superiority) to protect against their inner vulnerability and powerlessness. They try to restore a sense of control by dominating, making demands, and creating a sense of entitlement. A look at the lives of many dictators reveals childhoods marked by brutality, neglect, depression, and desperate attempts to compensate for this loss of control. Still others assume excessive responsibility to solve all the problems of the world in a futile attempt to prevent pain. The antidotes to this cause involve the development of empathy and compassion and a willingness to accept the world's imperfections.

5. *Social environment.* In the workplace, escalating expectations, lack of personal attention, and competition among individuals tend to promote anger by increasing the feelings of inadequacy or being unacceptable. Increasing media violence also encourages anger and aggression. So-called "reality television talk shows" tend to desensitize the viewer to suffering. It is not surprising, therefore, that children laugh at others' suffering or think that it is acceptable to resolve conflict with violence and insults. Increasingly, we see more examples of vulgarity, exploitation, and misanthropy, not only in the media, but in the workplace, the locker room, and the home. Connections to others have historically tended to keep a lid on aggression. However, the decline of family, neighborhood, and religious communities in recent years makes aggression more commonplace.

6. *Skill deficits.* Some people have simply not yet learned the skills of anger management: conflict resolution, problem solving, humor, constructive ways to gain power/attention, self-control, empathy, compassion, and tolerance. In "adult-free" homes, some children have not been taught limits and the rules of living. (Relative to previous generations, today's children are more likely to live in homes where there is only one parent or to be "latchkey children," unsupervised because one or both parents are away working.) All of these skills are readily learnable.

7. *Biology.* The mind and body are connected. The state of the body therefore exerts a great influence on our feelings. It is said that fatigue makes cowards of us all. Given the relationship between fear and anger, it becomes critical to have adequate rest and physical conditioning. Likewise, conditions such as hunger, poor nutrition, noise, shift work, insomnia, and temperature extremes need to be considered. Alcohol masks anger but does not regulate it. Therefore, the influence of alcohol or any other substance can ultimately increase anger and aggression.

Your physiological reactivity is determined to a great degree by the state of your nervous system. In many people, the nervous system has been sensitized by stressful experiences. This means that the structure and function of the neurons have changed in such a way that they overreact to smaller provocations. We now understand that cortisol, one of the hormones secreted in response to stress, especially the loss of control, can shrink a part of the brain called the hippocampus. The hippocampus helps the brain store memories with appropriate emotions. So excessively angry memories coupled with the habit of anger keep the nervous system sensitized. Fortunately, hippocampi that have been damaged by cortisol can be restored by a number of the approaches suggested in this book, including exercise and cognitive restructuring.

Some people seem to be genetically prone to overreact neurologically. However, this appears to be only a minority influence that can be offset by the acquisition of anger management skills. Finally, a shortage of serotonin appears to increase reactivity to stressors. Serotonin is a neurotransmitter, or a chemical that plays an important role in conveying messages in the brain. Sometimes serotonin-enhancing medication can lessen the tendency toward aggression and anger.

8. *Too little time for inner peace and recreation.* As the pace of living increases, there is less time to nurture oneself spiritually. This leads to a type of pain that can be expressed by frustration, irritation, and other forms of anger.

9. *Mental or medical illness.* Anger is a symptom of numerous mental illnesses. When these mental illnesses exist, the care of a com-

petent mental health professional is needed. These mental illnesses include post-traumatic stress disorder, schizophrenia, depression, anxiety, substance abuse, complicated grief, personality disorders (borderline, antisocial, narcissistic),[2] and brain injury.[3] Likewise, medical illnesses, including seizures, toxicities, hormonal imbalances, tumors, hypoglycemia, and chronic pain warrant a full medical evaluation.

When Is Anger a Problem?

As we discussed, anger is a universal emotion. It is not always bad. Anger can occasionally be useful if (1) the intent is to help or elevate (i.e., when anger leads to personal growth, lifts or protects oneself or others, or stops destructive treatment); or (2) the anger is measured, controlled, and leads to constructive actions (improved concentration, motivation, and performance). *Useful anger is devoid of malice, hatred, or hostile aggression.*

For example, no relationship grows without mutual respect and limits, so constructive anger might lead one to firmly and calmly assert: "I won't stand for disrespectful treatment from anybody—not even you."[4] The person then leaves the room, allowing the offender to be alone with his or her conscience. Here the person addresses the problem without demeaning the other person. Or, one's computer illiteracy might irritate one enough to finally master that computer. Here the energy is directed toward personal growth, not destruction of the computer.

Problem Anger

Intends to hurt, punish, disparage, or avenge, rather than to build, protect, or defend

Contains malice, hatred, or hostile aggression

Is excessive (disproportionate to the offense) or out of control

Is too frequent, too intense, or lasts too long

Is badly timed

Keeps you constantly on edge, irritable, cynical, cold, critical, or sarcastic

Is chronic

Harms yourself, others, or relationships; leads you to do foolish things

Is marked by cruel behavior, including verbal, physical, or emotional abuse, and cruelty to animals

Does not feel good; destroys peace; causes you significant distress

Impairs performance (driving, job, relationship, thinking, memory, judgment, creativity; e.g., a soldier recklessly charges the enemy and gets shot)

Tries to control or manipulate others (e.g., demands good treatment or respect)

Is easily provoked; impulsive; pops out when you are not expecting it

Is marked by violence

Is argumentative; refuses to compromise; is quick to pick fights; needs to win the argument rather than resolve the problem; needs to be right—because being wrong makes one feel worthless

Blames others for your own problems

Leads to power struggles

Is needed to avoid depression or to feel confident

Is used to dominate others or get your way

Leads to behaviors that you later feel ashamed of

Makes others feel diminished

Takes a toll on loved ones; makes them uncomfortable

Leads you to play the martyr; suffer silently

Is evidenced by having few friends or social skills—sharing, waiting turns, tolerating minor faults

Assumes people's motives are to harm you

Leads to nothing productive—is expressed in destructive ways rather than asserting, problem solving, or talking it over

Can't overlook relatively minor mistakes of self or others; is uncomfortable with imperfections

Leads to excessive smoking, alcohol, drugs, gambling, caffeine, sex, exercise, shopping, or work to sedate the anger or underlying pain

Covers deeper feelings and needs (insecurity, loneliness, low self-esteem, etc.)

Antagonizes others

Obstructs the reasonable progress of others

The Pros and Cons of Anger

Despite the obvious costs of anger, we still get angry. Why? Because anger is a habit that feels so justified and has many apparent, immediate rewards. If there were no rewards, we would cease to become angry. If anger seems to have worked for you in the past, it might be very difficult to give it up or reduce it. Thus, before trying to change something that has worked for you, let's do what a manager might do when asked to change a successful practice: a cost–benefit analysis. On a sheet of paper list all the advantages of anger; then list all the disadvantages. Before you start, try to visualize the short- and long-term effects of anger on yourself. Then imagine the consequences of your anger to others. Imagine their feelings when exposed to your anger.

When you are finished, look below at the responses other people have given.

Advantages

The benefits of getting angry are . . .

Energizes (I get an adrenaline rush)

Sharpens my faculties, focus, and concentration

Sense of power and control

Gains compliance in the short term (e.g., I yell at the kids and they quiet down for a little while)

Deadens my fear

Minimizes my feeling of inadequacy for a time

Helps me stand up for good causes

Alerts me that something is wrong, that I'm not getting what I want

Motivates me to change a personal weakness, develop inner strength

Prods me to leave an abusive situation

Gains respect, attention, fear

I'm seen as superior

Points out societal and personal wrongs, and motivates me to change them

Defends my ego against guilt, fear, grief, hurt, pain, helplessness, sadness ("He's the problem, not me.")

Vents frustration, releases tension

Protects me

Helps me know what I want

Expresses myself; my will to live and excel

Gives me a sense of self (some people feel emotionally dead, but anger is one feeling that might be okay and makes them feel alive)

Makes me feel that I'm right

Bonds me with others who are angry at the same thing

Gets my way

Disadvantages

The costs of getting angry are . . .

I dislike the feeling of being out of control

I'm viewed negatively by others; creates a bad impression

Getting even consumes energy

Fatiguing, draining, burns me out

Makes me look ugly

Escalates my own anger

Activates anger in others (our feelings tend to create similar feelings in others)

Instigates aggression, retaliation, and sabotage by others

Deadens the true feelings that are underneath my anger—both good and bad

Does not influence others in a lasting way, but only for the short term

Disrupts, distracts me from performing my best

Interferes with problem solving

Impairs judgment

I'm learning to distrust more and more people (Near death, Stalin told Khrushchev, "I trust no one, not even myself.")[5]

People dislike me, distrust me, resent me, avoid me, are cool to me, see me as mean

Alienates others, sours relationships

Decreases goodwill, trust, satisfaction, and enjoyment in relationships

Causes people to avoid giving me potentially useful feedback because of fear

May lead to my aggressing against or abusing weaker individuals (violence, assault, rape)

Could get me in legal trouble (jailed for violence, road rage)

Leads to conflict with others

Is causing me to withdraw from or avoid others

Damage to property

The angrier I am generally, the more prone I am to further provocations

Derails my career plans, gets me fired (e.g., Patton, Nixon)

Leads to taking on hated characteristics of others (arrogance, bullying, prejudice, judging)

Long-term health problems. Those prone to anger, hostility, and/or aggression are at higher risk for high blood pressure, coronary heart disease, stroke, death from all causes, and job injuries. They might be at greater risk for headaches, backaches, cancer, ulcers, and gastrointestinal disturbance. They are more likely to smoke and relapse from psychological illness. In post-traumatic stress disorder, anger hinders the processing of trauma and is associated with symptom severity following exposure to traumatic events. People who are prone to anger tend to oversecrete stress hormones (cortisol and catecholamines), which damage heart muscles and the cells lining blood vessels, make blood platelets stickier, weaken the immune system, and raise cholesterol. Disrupted relationships and loneliness are also associated with greater risk of heart disease.

Robs me of happiness, joy, peace, and harmony with others

Takes a toll on loved ones

Memories are irritating rather than pleasant

Destroys pleasure (e.g., driving used to be a beautiful adventure when I was a child; now it has become a heated battle)

Blocks healing because I don't acknowledge and feel the deep hurts

I don't take responsibility for changing my behavior or healing my weaknesses, so I never discover all my strengths; no self-scrutiny, so there's no growth or change

I don't resolve underlying feelings—so anger remains

I don't learn that some people are trustworthy and kind— so anger reinforces mistrust

It can lead to unpleasant guilt

I'm setting a rotten example for my children

I hate the person I've become; damaged self-esteem

This exercise reveals that there are some significant advantages to anger. This is why it is so hard to release. Now ask yourself:

- Is anger a problem to me in terms of its costs? Is it to my advantage to get angry?

- Is the anger serving me in the long run? Is it helping me cope and function well? Get promoted? Be loved by my family? Get what I really want?
- Is this how I want to see myself? Be remembered?
- Are there other ways to feel powerful, secure, and adequate, and to meet my goals without destructive anger?
- What are the ways to be less angry and more productive and satisfied?

Before moving on, please consider the positive consequences of being less angry. Imagine what your life would be like if you were less angry. Some people have responded:

I'll be viewed as a nonjudgmental, level-headed person.

I'll probably be more liked, trusted, and respected by other people, rather than feared.

I'll be more predictable.

I'll feel more in control of my emotions.

I'll feel more relaxed.

I'll feel more comfortable with myself.

I'll influence people more effectively, through leadership, negotiation, and respect, rather than fear and intimidation.

My cholesterol and blood pressure will likely drop.

I'll function more logically.

I'll be more productive by reclaiming the energy I usually spend on anger.

I'll have more energy.

I'll experience less guilt and more self-respect.

I'll be more attractive and peaceful.

Where Are We Going?
The Opposites of Anger

It is often said that sick people have the fewest options. Let's spend a few moments recognizing our choices. The most effective problem solvers are extremely creative. They not only recognize the problem, but they can conceive many solutions to the problem and various pathways to those solutions. If anger is the problem, then it benefits us to know as many alternatives to anger as possible.

When teaching at the Pentagon, I once explained that Type A behavior is the readiness to be angry. I then asked the group of participants to describe the opposites of readiness to be angry. One conscientious Type A Army officer responded, "The readiness not to be angry." I replied, "That is neutral, but what is the *opposite*?" He bore down, furrowed his brow in thought, and responded more loudly, "The readiness *not* to be angry!" A bright and successful woman, who was ending her third marriage, then said almost plaintively, "Maybe that's our problem. We can't conceive the opposites."

What do you think are the opposites of anger? The more you can identify, the better. List as many anger opposites as you can on a sheet of paper. When you have finished, check your responses against those that others have given.

The opposite of the readiness to be angry is the readiness to . . .

- Be a peacemaker
- Forebear (refrain, exercise self-control under provocation)
- Tolerate others' imperfections, pain, difficulties
- Respect others, their rights and views
- See all as equals
- Empathize, understand others' viewpoints
- Accept
- Be compassionate
- Enjoy lifting others' burdens
- Cooperate
- Think in terms of "we" rather than "me" so much
- Be unperturbed

- Be nonreactive, indifferent
- Laugh at mistakes
- Be optimistic
- Be vulnerable
- Be flexible
- Be kindhearted
- Be friendly
- Harmonize
- Be conciliatory
- Be happy, content
- Compromise
- Be strong, secure
- Be benevolent
- Have inner peace
- Be calm
- Love
- Have goodwill, trust
- Comfort
- Be patient
- Compliment
- Be secure inside
- Really feel all emotions
- Be sensitive
- Enjoy myself, have fun
- Operate from a service motive, rather than a status motive

Considering the many opposites of anger, we see that there are many bright possibilities ahead—many constructive, satisfying goals to strive for. *Managing anger certainly goes well beyond simply reducing anger. It takes us to a calmer, more peaceful existence—one that is within our reach.*

What Can I Expect?

Anger *can* be managed! Much research has shown that people with excessive anger can significantly and fairly quickly decrease it through the approaches described in this sourcebook.[6] You will learn skills that address all of the important levels: thoughts, images, attitudes, and behaviors. With regular practice, you can expect to maintain and improve upon your gains.

The goal of this program is not to eliminate anger altogether, but to help you gain control over it. In other words, to manage anger. This means:

- Reducing general levels of anger
- Decreasing the intensity, duration, and frequency of angry episodes
- Keeping anger from escalating too fast or beyond appropriate levels so that you can function at your best

Anger management does not mean bottling up anger. This can lead to explosive anger. Rather, it means that we acknowledge the normal feelings of anger that arise, and learn to appropriately defuse and express them.

This book aims to preserve and enhance your strong qualities, not to change your basic nature. Some people wonder, "Will managing anger make me weak, a wimp, or less effective as a leader?" To address such questions, a study was undertaken at the U.S. Army War College. The War College trains future generals, the best and the brightest leaders in the Army. Pentagon officials had decided to implement a course to reduce Type A behavior in an attempt to reduce the number of heart attacks that afflicted so many of these officers in their most productive years. Type As are people who are hostile, angry, competitive, and in a hurry. While reducing Type A behavior was known to reduce the risk of heart attack, there was concern that teaching officers to manage anger might make them less effective as leaders. So researchers measured changes in these officers as a result of the course. Findings indicated that the officers became more effective leaders, not worse, in all aspects measured. For example, the officers reported that they performed better, being better able to listen to others and set wise priorities. Their judgment, understanding of others, humor, and self-esteem improved. They also enjoyed their relationships with others more.[7] As we used to teach at the Pentagon, it is not Type A behavior that gets people ahead, but competence. Type As and Type Bs can be equally ambitious. However, the motives are very different. Type Bs pursue excellence because it is enjoyable, not to prove their worth. The pur suit arises from a foundation of inner security, not hostility or competition. With less hostility, careers are less likely to be derailed, as happened to several famous Type As, including the brilliant WWII general George Patton and former president Richard M. Nixon.

Research and experience show that people can learn to regulate anger reasonably quickly. For example, in one study, hyperactive, impulsive boys fairly quickly learned to withstand verbal taunts. They watched others stay calm and learned to tell themselves things like, "I'm not going to let them get to me. Stay calm."[8] Also, the Treating Type A Behavior program at the Pentagon halved hostility in the Department of the Army employees and officers in just four weeks.[9]

It is reasonable to expect that learning anger management skills will improve your health and possibly prevent or delay the onset of disease, especially in those who are at risk for cardiovascular diseases. Cardiovascular disease is the number one killer in America, accounting for somewhat less than half of all deaths. By comparison, cancer, the second-leading killer, accounts for approximately half as many deaths. Over twenty studies[10] have shown that combinations of the techniques taught here (relaxation, stress management, diet, exercise, connecting to others) significantly reduce hostility, second heart attacks, blood pressure, heart rate, and/or levels of cholesterol in the blood. You can also expect to acquire many of the opposites of anger discussed previously, making life more peaceful and enjoyable.

Mastering anger is not easy, nor is it learned once and for all. Rather, the process involves the acquisition of new principles and skills, and the reinforcement of these principles and skills through regular practice. The program described will take you about seven weeks to work through. It is recommended that you practice the skills as you go, since simply reading about skills is not the same as acquiring and mastering them; think of an athlete trying to learn a sport without practice. Although challenging, the process is straightforward and growth is within reach of every individual.

The Different Ways Anger Manifests

Being able to name anger and recognize its diverse forms of expression is the first step to managing it. We suggest that you try this powerful activity before analyzing its very important purpose. On a sheet of paper, make three columns. In the first column, list as many feeling words as you can for anger. In the second, list as many metaphors as you can that describe anger (e.g., flipped my lid). In the third column, list as many behaviors as you can that show anger. When finished, check Table 1.1 to see if there are some you missed.

Table 1.1 Varieties of Anger

This table lists the wide-ranging varieties of anger: feeling words, metaphors, and behaviors. Notice the choices.

Feeling Words	Metaphors	Behaviors
aggravated	angry enough to kill you/	accusing, pointing, or shaking finger
agitated	shoot you/cut you off/	aggression
angry	cry/strangle you/	argue
annoyed	explode	attack posture, body tightens,
belligerent	bent out of shape	forward lean
bitter	blew a fuse/gasket/my top	avoid eye contact, look away
churning	blind with rage	backbite
cranky	blood boiling	become quiet, cold shoulder, silent
cross	boiling mad	treatment
defensive	breathing fire	blaming
disappointed	burning mad	bullying
embittered	couldn't see straight	clench fist/jaw/teeth, furrowed brow,
enraged	fighting mad	frown
exasperated	fight waiting to happen	competitiveness
frustrated	fit to be tied	criticism, put-downs, sniping
fuming	flipped/freaked out	cry
furious	flipped his wig	damage/destroy property
grouchy	flying off the handle	demanding
hate	going ballistic/postal	denial
hostile	got up on the wrong side	drink, use drugs
hot	of the bed	fantasizing harm to offender
hurt	had a cow	fight back
ill-tempered	hit the ceiling/roof	glare, looks that could kill
impatient	hopping mad	harassment
incensed	hotheaded	insults, name-calling
indignant	hot potato	interrupt others

Table 1.1 (Continued)

Feeling Words	Metaphors	Behaviors
infuriated	hot under the collar, hot	make demands
insulted	as a firecracker	nagging
irate	icy cold	physical arousal (flushed face, increas-
irked	in a snit	ed heart rate and blood pressure,
irritable	loaded and ready to fire	rapid eye blinks, darting eyes, rapid
irritated	losing my cool	breathing, restless, sweaty, etc.)
livid	mad as a bat out of hell	physically attack or harm (hit, batter,
mad	madder than a mad hatter	grab, shake, push)
malicious	madder than a wet hen	pout
miffed	madder than a wet hornet	raise voice, shout
offended	madder than hell	retaliate physically or verbally
out of control	meltdown	roll eyes
outraged	on the warpath	sarcastic comment, hostile humor
peeved	outside/beside herself	scold
perturbed	popped his cork	scowl, grimace, snarl
pissed off (royally)	raging bull/maniac	seek revenge (e.g., spread rumors)
rage	ready to explode	sit on horn, or other aggressive
raving	red hot	driving behavior
resentful	saw red	slam door, phone, etc.
revengeful	seeing red	sneer
riled up	short fuse	sulk
seething	simmering	teach a lesson
slamming	sizzling	teasing
spiteful	slow burn	temper tantrum
steamed, steaming	smoke coming out of ears	threats (verbal, gestures,
teed/ticked off	so angry I could	intimidation, etc.)
upset	explode/bust	throws things
uptight	so angry I couldn't speak	uncooperative/disruptive
vengeful	so angry I could spit	vulgar language or gestures
vexed	spitting nails	walk or turn away, storm out,
volatile	steaming mad	withdraw
violent	went through the roof	whine, moan, complain
worked up	wigged out	yell

Next, draw an anger thermometer like the one in Figure 1.1. From your list of anger words, select four each for low, medium, and high levels of anger. Then rank these according to their intensity within each group. Write these words alongside the thermometer.

Figure 1.1 Anger Thermometer

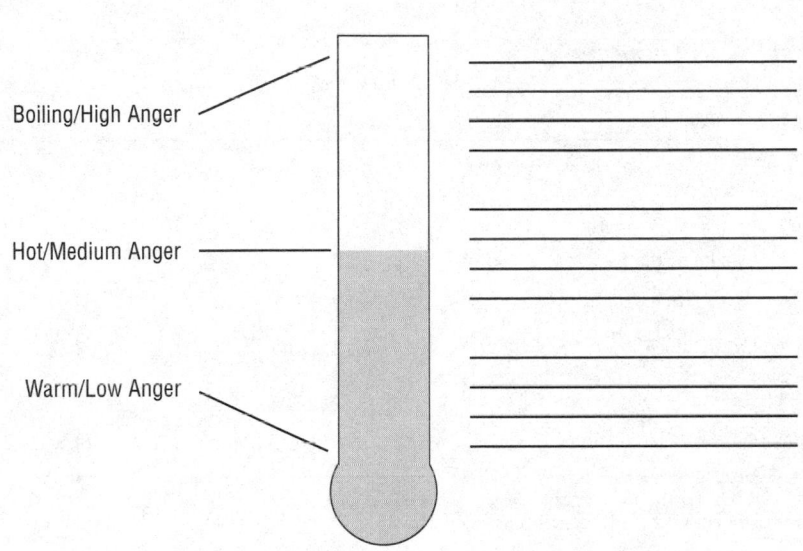

These activities accomplish three important purposes. First, recognizing the gradations of anger shows that anger is not an all-or-nothing phenomenon. It suggests that we can regulate it, tuning anger up or down. Second, developing an anger vocabulary allows one to verbalize—to say, "I'm getting frustrated"—before anger boils over or is expressed destructively. Third, they help us to realize that the metaphors and behaviors that we sometimes use really reflect authentic feelings that need to be addressed, perhaps in new ways.

Assessing the Proneness to Anger

The assessment presented in Exhibit 1.2, the Anger Checkup, will help you get a better sense of the way you experience and express anger. Circle the responses that best apply to you. Most of the value of the Anger Checkup lies in the process of completing it and gaining insights about yourself. Be as objective and honest as you can, without judging yourself. Remember that everyone gets angry at times. Calm, nonjudgmental awareness is the first step in managing anger. The scoring key at the end will give you a rough idea of what your score means.

Exhibit 1.2 The Anger Checkup

Part I: Anger Experience

I generally feel . . .	Almost Never	Sometimes	Often	Almost Always
1. Angry	1	2	3	4
2. Irritated, bothered by a lot of things	1	2	3	4
3. Easily provoked	1	2	3	4
4. Impatient	1	2	3	4
5. Resentful	1	2	3	4
6. Jealous	1	2	3	4
7. Grouchy	1	2	3	4
8. Unhappy	1	2	3	4

Describes me:	Not at All	A Little	Moderately Well	Very Well
9. I get angry often (*frequency*).	1	2	3	4
10. It takes me a long time to calm down when I get angry (*duration*).	1	2	3	4
11. I've felt angry for a long time.	1	2	3	4
12. Resentments are mounting.	1	2	3	4
13. When angry, I'm unreasonable or out of control.	1	2	3	4
14. I blow up quickly (fly off the handle).	1	2	3	4
15. I'm hotheaded.	1	2	3	4
16. People may not know it, but I burn inside when I'm angry.	1	2	3	4
17. It is difficult to overlook peoples' mistakes or shortcomings.	1	2	3	4

I get angry when . . .	Strongly Disagree	Disagree	Agree	Strongly Agree
18. Others disagree with me or challenge me.	1	2	3	4
19. I'm interrupted.	1	2	3	4
20. I'm delayed, or kept waiting.	1	2	3	4
21. People let me down.	1	2	3	4
22. People show weaknesses or make mistakes.	1	2	3	4
23. I'm criticized or humiliated.	1	2	3	4
24. I don't get the recognition or respect I deserve.	1	2	3	4
25. I get behind the wheel.	1	2	3	4
26. I'm not loved.	1	2	3	4
27. I'm ignored.	1	2	3	4
28. Things don't go the way I want.	1	2	3	4
29. People have annoying habits.	1	2	3	4
30. There isn't enough time to do all I want to do.	1	2	3	4
31. I fail to meet my goals.	1	2	3	4

Total Score—Part I (items 1–31) _____

Part II: Attitudes (hostility, cynicism, enmity)

	Strongly Disagree	Disagree	Agree	Strongly Agree
32. People are selfish, deceitful, exploitive—they just want to use you and can't be trusted.	1	2	3	4
33. I tend to nurse grudges.	1	2	3	4
34. I like to get even or seek revenge.	1	2	3	4
35. I'm safer if I don't trust people.	1	2	3	4

Part II: Attitudes (hostility, cynicism, enmity) (continued)

	Strongly Disagree	Disagree	Agree	Strongly Agree
36. Most people have an angle and will hurt you if you let them.	1	2	3	4
37. I expect people to screw me if given the chance.	1	2	3	4
38. Most people don't like me.	1	2	3	4
39. I don't like or trust too many people.	1	2	3	4
40. I regard people with contempt.	1	2	3	4
41. There are people I strongly dislike.	1	2	3	4
42. I feel the need to compete, dominate others, be stronger, or control others.	1	2	3	4
43. I don't enjoy others' accomplishments or successes.	1	2	3	4
44. Few people get close to me.	1	2	3	4
45. I tend to distrust people's motives.	1	2	3	4
46. I have a large or growing list of people to avoid.	1	2	3	4
47. In general, I feel negatively toward certain groups of people (e.g., certain races, age groups, etc.).	1	2	3	4
48. A lot of people remind me of people I don't like.	1	2	3	4
49. I'm afraid that people will reject me if I let them really know me.	1	2	3	4
50. I feel like hurting people.	1	2	3	4
51. I don't feel remorse for hurting people.	1	2	3	4

	Strongly Disagree	Disagree	Agree	Strongly Agree
52. I distrust people who are friendly.	1	2	3	4
53. I imagine (hope, or would like to see) people getting what they deserve.	1	2	3	4
54. People are only nice to you in order to get something.	1	2	3	4

Total Score—Part II (items 32–54) _____

Part III: Behaviors (aggression, exploding, violence, verbal attacks)

I . . .	Almost Never	Sometimes	Often	Almost Always
55. Withdraw, keep my distance from people.	1	2	3	4
56. Become uncooperative, disruptive, interfere with others' plans.	1	2	3	4
57. Don't show my feelings (e.g., sadness, vulnerability), except for anger.	1	2	3	4
58. Am overly competitive, need to beat others, must win.	1	2	3	4
59. Argue, pick fights, have repeating conflicts.	1	2	3	4
60. Watch people, keep an eye on them to make sure they're doing what they should.	1	2	3	4
61. Have to be right, win arguments.	1	2	3	4
62. Scold, berate, put people in their places.	1	2	3	4
63. Use obscenities or vulgar language when I speak.	1	2	3	4
64. Complain frequently.	1	2	3	4

Part III: Behaviors (aggression, exploding, violence, verbal attacks) (continued)

I . . .	Almost Never	Sometimes	Often	Almost Always
65. Dominate, bully, threaten.	1	2	3	4
66. Fight back, retaliate.	1	2	3	4
67. Am unfriendly to people.	1	2	3	4
68. End friendships quickly (e.g., when people disappoint me).	1	2	3	4
69. Use sarcasm, teasing, mocking jokes.	1	2	3	4
70. Use humor as a put-down—not to share common pains.	1	2	3	4
71. Am critical, and use put-downs or call people names.	1	2	3	4
72. Manage people through compulsion or intimidation.	1	2	3	4
73. Am unforgiving and spiteful.	1	2	3	4
74. Use painkillers (or drugs, alcohol, sex, TV, food, work, sleep, shopping) to kill emotional pain.	1	2	3	4
75. Keep others away from me (through anger, obesity, poor hygiene; or through boisterous, crude, or cold behavior).	1	2	3	4
76. Seek ways to get even, take revenge.	1	2	3	4
77. Show rage when things don't go my way, or I'm under great pressure.	1	2	3	4
78. Have angry outbursts, (tantrums, switch from calm to angry, blow up).	1	2	3	4

I . . .	Almost Never	Sometimes	Often	Almost Always
79. Blame others for my problems (scapegoat).	1	2	3	4
80. Become violent (hit, push, shake, grab, throw things, destroy property, slam doors, drive dangerously or too fast).	1	2	3	4
81. Become verbally abusive —saying nasty, mean things.	1	2	3	4
82. Yell, scream.	1	2	3	4
83. Speak loudly (as a way to keep control) or abruptly.	1	2	3	4
84. Interrupt others to finish their sentences, hurrying their speech.	1	2	3	4
85. Tend to antagonize, rather than get along with others.	1	2	3	4
86. Force sex on an unwilling partner.	1	2	3	4
87. Nag.	1	2	3	4
88. Make accusations (e.g., "Why are you so defensive?").	1	2	3	4
89. Like to intimidate or make people afraid of me.	1	2	3	4
90. Shift conversations to the faults of others (younger generations, bosses, corporations, etc.).	1	2	3	4
91. Cry when angry.	1	2	3	4
92. Have difficulty relaxing or enjoying life's loveliness.	1	2	3	4
93. Defend or justify my anger.	1	2	3	4

Total Score—Part III (55–93) _____

Part IV: Physical Arousal

When angry, I experience . . .	Almost Never	Sometimes	Often	Almost Always
94. Flushed face.	1	2	3	4
95. Increased heart rate or pounding heart.	1	2	3	4
96. Increased blood pressure.	1	2	3	4
97. Rapid eye blinks.	1	2	3	4
98. Darting eyes.	1	2	3	4
99. Rapid breathing, sighs, or gasping for breath.	1	2	3	4
100. Sweating.	1	2	3	4
101. Facial displays—furrowed brow, frown, scowl, or glare.	1	2	3	4
102. Attack posture—forward lean, pointing or shaking finger.	1	2	3	4
103. Clenched fist.	1	2	3	4
104. Clenched teeth.	1	2	3	4
105. Facial tautness—especially around jaw, eyes, forehead.	1	2	3	4
106. Tight muscles.	1	2	3	4

Total Score—Part IV (94–106) _____

Part V: Significant Other Report

Have a spouse or someone else who knows you very well (preferably someone who lives with you) complete the Anger Checkup about you. Note the differences.

Anger Checkup Scoring Key

	Low Anger	Moderate Anger	High Anger
Part I	31–43	44–65	66–124
Part II	23–32	33–48	49–92
Part III	39–55	56–82	83–156
Part IV	13–18	19–27	28–52

Other Ways of Assessing Anger

Rate your anger mastery on a percentage scale: _____%

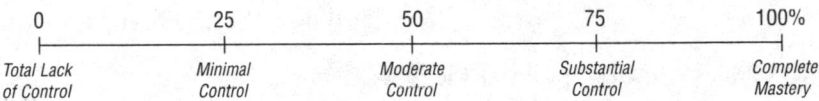

0	25	50	75	100%
Total Lack of Control	Minimal Control	Moderate Control	Substantial Control	Complete Mastery

In your daily activities, how often do you feel that anger keeps you from doing what you want, or causes you to do something you do not want to do? _____

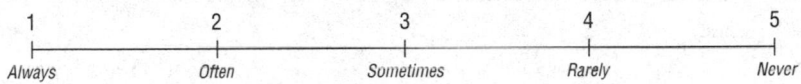

1	2	3	4	5
Always	Often	Sometimes	Rarely	Never

How serious is your problem with anger? _____

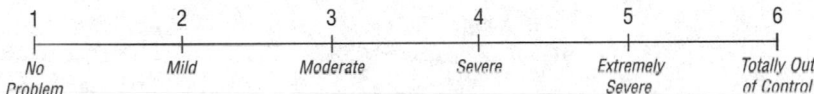

1	2	3	4	5	6
No Problem	Mild	Moderate	Severe	Extremely Severe	Totally Out of Control

Drills

- Look for signs of hostility on television and in movies.
- Notice humorous jokes and bumper stickers. Note if they are hostile.
- Notice signs of anger/hostility in others.
- Notice signs of anger/hostility in yourself.
- Identify your hooks. Pay attention to your reactions— thoughts, emotions, physical changes, behaviors.
- Ask a loved one to identify signs of anger in yourself.

Reflections

No man is angry that feels not himself hurt.

(Francis Bacon, *Essays*, "Of Anger," 1625)

I've never known a mean person who wasn't in pain.

> (Anonymous)

We become what we hate.

> (William Irwin Thompson)

Cynics are disappointed idealists.

> (Ingrid Bengis)

Anger is never without a reason, but seldom with a good one.

> (Benjamin Franklin, *Poor Richard's Almanac*, 1754)

Anger is "the chief enemy of public happiness and private peace."

> (Hyman Meltzer)[11]

Every minute you're angry is sixty seconds of unhappiness.

> (Anonymous)

Suggested Activity

Start keeping a journal that describes your hooks and the various ways you react to them.

2

The Principles of Anger Management

If we could read the secret histories of our enemies we should find sorrow and suffering enough to disarm all hostility.

—Longfellow

Managing Anger

Learning to manage anger is both liberating and empowering, although it is rarely an easy or quick process. With patient and persistent practice, however, the way you experience and express anger can be greatly modified. The following important principles will guide you on your journey toward anger mastery and greater emotional intelligence.

Realize That Anger Is a Choice

Anger is a choice. We choose to have more or less of it. No one makes us angry. The world presents challenges, and we are responsible for how we react to these challenges—not others, not the world, not our parents. We choose whom or what we let get under our skin. We decide whether or not we'll get angry, how much anger to generate, how and when to express it, how long to hold on to it, and whether it will be constructive or destructive. If you don't believe that, think of times when you stopped yourself from flying off at your boss or a police officer. We decide whether or not to let resentment take up residence in our minds. We can choose to talk calmly rather than scream or become violent. We can walk away from a fight rather than become embroiled in conflict. We can wait until we cool off to address a sensitive topic, especially if the other person is feeling defensive, angry, or distracted.

Sometimes it helps to realize that problem anger does not gain us the power, control, respect, or love we want. It only makes us more powerless by placing our peace in the hands of someone or something else. It drives people away. In short, we put ourselves in the powerless victim role.

Rather than blaming others or trying to fix them, it is often more fruitful to think, "Part of the problem is . . . (my readiness to hold people in contempt, my impatience, my unwillingness to accept imperfection or ambiguity)." This is more likely to help you see what adjustments will help you cope better. Chances are that we will not change people against their will, but we can choose to make our reactions more beautiful, and perhaps earn respect, cooperation, or love.

Tibetan teachers relate that a monk was once meditating outside of the monastery. A man walked by and asked what the monk was doing. The monk responded with irritation, "I'm cultivating patience." In other words, we need challenges to develop our strengths. Rather than viewing challenges negatively, we can view them gratefully, as great teachers.

You might ask yourself, "Will anger further my cause?" "Will I make myself miserable in the long run?" "Am I spending ten dollars on every nickel-and-dime problem?" "Is it possible to let go a bit and not try to control so much?" "Maybe the world won't end if I don't get my way, if I am not 100 percent efficient, or if someone dislikes me."

If you feel anger rising, try a distraction. Read, garden, or watch a movie. Try to forget about it. *Life is too short to get angry every time you have a right to.* We can accept that we don't always get our way, and that's okay. We can be persistent, determined, forceful, or persuasive; we can keep fighting for something beautiful or just, but not be angry. We can realize that we have many options that usually work better than anger. For example, we can post reasonable rules for our children and the consequences of breaking the rules, then calmly say, "You know the rules; you've chosen the consequences." If getting lost "makes you" crazy, you might buy a global positioning device. If the computer "drives you" mad, you might get needed help. We can try our earnest best, but not become too attached to the outcome. We cannot always control the outcome. We are not likely to change others. We *can* control ourselves.

Distinguish Disturbed from Nondisturbed Anger

Disturbed anger is out of control and disproportionate to the offense (e.g., rage, fury). It hurts ourselves and/or others and leads to nothing productive. Nondisturbed anger has a purpose: to bring about change for the good. It is measured, controlled, and leads to constructive actions. For example, we might take reasonable action to prevent disrespectful treatment or solve a problem through respectful communication. Nondisturbed anger is void of malice, hatred, resentments, or hostile aggression—and values the well-being of oneself and others.

As the Dalai Lama has taught,[1] occasionally anger can be useful if it leads to constructive action, if motivated by concern/compassion, or if there is a need to cleanse the system of pent up feelings by confiding. For example, if you let someone's harmful behavior go unchallenged, you might reinforce bad habits in the other. But anger with malice is never useful. Thus, you can correct with compassion, but without hatred. If you can correct the problem, why be angry? If you can't, why be angry? What is important enough to destroy your peace? The question really is not should we give up all anger, but can we choose when and how to experience it? One can forcefully pursue justice without bitterness or malice.

Understand That Attitudes Precede Skills

Whether we are exploring anger at home, at the workplace, in traffic, or in play, *attitudes of the heart underlie all of the important skills of anger management*. We shall explore three especially important attitudes: respect, compassion, and empathy.

The Special Attitude of Respect

When I was a cadet at West Point, it fell our lot to memorize numerous passages and facts that were recited as a means of instilling discipline, or imposing punishment. One particular passage turned out to be the greatest leadership lesson I ever learned. I am especially grateful for it, and have used it often in dealing with people that I have led. Although it speaks of leading soldiers, its wisdom is equally applicable to all human relationships. I recommend not only reading, but, if possible, memorizing it.

> The discipline which makes the soldiers of a free country reliable in battle is not to be gained by harsh or tyrannical treatment. On the contrary, such treatment is far more likely to destroy than to make an army. It is possible to impart instruction and to give commands in such a manner and such a tone of voice as to inspire in the soldier no feeling but an intense desire to obey, while the opposite manner and tone of voice cannot fail to excite strong resentment and a desire to disobey. The one mode or the other of dealing with subordinates springs from a corresponding spirit in the breast of the commander. He who feels the respect which is due to others cannot fail to inspire in them regard for himself, while he who feels, and hence manifests, disrespect toward others, especially his inferiors, cannot fail to inspire hatred against himself.
>
> (Major General John M. Schofield)[2]

Esteeming others as ourselves, and treating them as we would wish to be treated, tends to bring out the best in others. We can:

• Respect others by speaking softly and calmly—unlike Type As, who speak loudly, rapidly, and in a demanding way.

• Look people in the eye with a pleasant expression, and watch your own facial expressions when someone is getting upset.

• Use care in how you express your hurts (e.g., "I was hurt when you were late for our special dinner," rather than, "You selfish, irresponsible idiot.").

• Use care in your speech—avoiding offensive language, name-calling, contempt, and unkind comments to or about others.

Compassion and Empathy

One day at the Pentagon, I was asking a class to identify the opposites of anger. One gentleman thoughtfully replied, "Compassion." We were all impressed by the impact of his response. I went home and looked up the word. Compassion is a beautiful word meaning sorrow for the suffering of others and the urge to help; deep sympathy.

Compassionate people recognize that all people are alike in that we all desire happiness and wish to avoid suffering. They desire to alleviate suffering rather than maintain it.

A primary school student, Mark Dapper, wrote:

> Compassion is when you want to help another person who is hurting or going through hard times, or has made some mistakes. It's really caring for someone else.
>
> Compassion begins by paying attention to others and really looking around. When people feel bad or are in trouble, they usually feel sad and all alone. Being compassionate tells a person that you care and that he's not alone. . . . If you help somebody you are really serving and helping [God].
>
> If you see someone who doesn't have a friend, you should go talk to them. Even a little smile and "hello" is being compassionate.
>
> The world would be a better place if everyone would help each other and show compassion.

Empathy is seeing the other person's point of view and feeling what they are feeling. When someone hurts or disappoints us, empathy asks, "Why would someone behave or feel that way? What unhealed wounds, insecurities, or fears exist? What need are they trying to fulfill? How are they trying to protect themselves? How would I feel if I were in their shoes? Maybe they are troubled, unhappy, or having problems, just like me." Empathy understands that hostile people are hurting people; that people who willingly hurt others are not in their right/best mind. Understanding that pain usually drives hostile behavior, we are less likely to take offense. We are more likely to see the redeeming value in another and think, "I wonder if I can help." If a waitress appears rude, we might joke, "Has it been one of those days?" When other people make a decision that hurts or disappoints us, instead of choosing bitterness, we might try to see it from their viewpoint. Maybe:

- There's a consideration that I don't know about.
- Their circumstances changed.
- They didn't like something they saw.
- They had an honest change of heart.

If problem anger is the great destroyer, compassion is the great healer—the great antidote for the pain and hurt that underlies anger. We can first learn to have compassion for ourselves by thinking, "It's okay to feel hurt, frustrated, or upset." Feel the hurt, and then heal it with loving kindness. When you stumble, be patient and kind, for this is your first time through this life. *The power to heal our own hurts comes from compassion. It does not come from demanding that others change their behavior*. First, others may not choose to comply with our demands, and even if they do, this does not address the real need. Later in the book we shall explore various approaches to heal inner wounds, soothe ourselves, and strengthen ourselves inwardly.

It is also very empowering to learn to apply compassion to others, even if we disapprove of their behaviors. A large Marine officer at the Pentagon related that he had recently been cut off by a driver. So he quickly passed the other driver, stopped at a light, and got out and screamed at him. I asked him how that felt. The officer replied,

"I felt ridiculous. Here I'm screaming at this little wimpy guy who is shaking and quivering." He accepted an assignment. The next time that happened he looked into the face of the driver and tried to see him as a fallible, suffering human being, who is just like he is. He said, "It was amazing how calm I remained." Another woman screamed, "How could my (deceased) father repeatedly rape me when he said he loved me." She came to realize that it was because he did not know how to relate normally to people, and not to hurt her. Although this realization in no way excused the behavior, understanding helped to neutralize much of the anger that had burdened her for years. Impatience thinks, "There is no excuse." Compassion and empathy reply, "Yes, there is—it's that people are imperfect and still learning."

Become a Serious Student of Peace

Seriously observe calm "copers." Ask them what they're thinking and how they handle their hooks. Notice how your anger ruins your peace. Ask others how they feel when you are angry (disliked, afraid, intimidated, put off, resentful). Anticipate hooks and ponder how you could handle them without undue anger. Watch yourself speaking to or about others. Does your speech contain cynicism, sarcasm, bitterness, or gossip? Associate with people who are peaceful, calm, and compassionate. Read about people who model the opposites of anger. (See the resources listed in Appendix B.)

Pay Attention to Your True Feelings

When we understand what the deeper hurts are, then we can address the deeper needs that feed the anger. Ask yourself what is underneath the anger. Label and express that feeling, be it frustration, powerlessness, inadequacy, rejection, sadness, fear, isolation, etc. Instead of blaming or trying to fix the other person, think: "At least some of the problem is . . . (e.g., my readiness to let someone make me feel devalued)." This will help you gain control over what you can control—yourself. Keep an anger journal to better understand underlying feelings and hurts.

Become More Resilient and Less Vulnerable

When someone reminds you of a flaw, think: "Oh right—I have a flaw. That's okay." Pat yourself on the back when you do a reasonably good job, and be as compassionate to yourself as you are to others. You might think of a peace shield, a light surrounding you and deflecting the barbs that could destroy your peace.

Minimize Contact with Provocations

Decrease exposure to media aggression/violence, which reinforces the tendency to react aggressively. As much as possible, minimize contact with people who are "stress carriers." You might stop seeing the person who chronically keeps you waiting.

Learn People Skills

- If you must correct or disagree with others, do it in a straightforward way, then be friendly afterward so that they know you don't harbor resentment.
- Try your best, speak honestly and from the heart, and don't get attached to the outcome.
- Change demands of imperfect people to requests/proposals. "It would be nice if you'd . . . ," "Would you please . . . "
- Assert yourself:

  - "Please don't criticize/tease me. I don't like that."
  - "Why would you want to say something that hurtful?"
  - "Nobody likes to feel stupid. How would you feel if I treated you that way?"

Use Humor

Humor is a special, important skill that will be explored in Chapter 14.

Attend to Your Physical and Spiritual Needs

Physical and spiritual needs will be explored in some detail in Chapters 9 and 16.

Step Back and Remember the Big Picture

To endure suffering with calmness, remember your ultimate purpose, which is long-term spiritual growth, inner peace, and happiness. Decide in advance not to destroy your own peace with anger. Scale back some expectations, since much anger comes from unrealistic expectations. We aren't perfect, why should we expect others to be? We haven't got everything all figured out. Why should we be surprised when others don't? Don't expect others to change, certainly not quickly. Don't be surprised by others' imperfections. Tim had patiently petitioned the Army for compensation for an illness acquired while on duty. Despite numerous bureaucratic frustrations, he reflected, "Bureaucrats are people who are sometimes ignorant of what they're supposed to be doing. In the Army there are a lot of people like that. You never win with anger." He patiently persisted, with help from many who admired his patience and character.

Reexamine your motives for working. If your ultimate goal is status, your ego will be on the line and easily hurt. However, if you make service your motive, your focus will be on elevating others and you'll be less likely to anger. General George C. Marshall understood this principle. Politicians during WWII wanted to decorate this highly respected and dedicated officer. However, he declined their awards because "receiving any decorations while our men were in the jungles of New Guinea or the isles of the Pacific especially or anywhere else there was heavy fighting . . . would not at all appear well."[3] He was more concerned with others than with himself. If our motive is to lift, serve, or love others, we can better tolerate ingratitude, mistreatment, and differences. We more readily compromise, apologize, and empathize.

Release, Release, Release

Let go of anger, bitterness, hatred, hostility, and resentment at every opportunity so that you can live with more peace. Try to forgive often. Don't torture yourself by reliving angry memories. Don't rant and rave or dwell on life's unfairness. Rather than fuming if you are kept waiting, bring a book to read and utilize that time well.

Although rage expresses caring and the will to live, the will to live is awakened much more strongly by love. Love preserves and expands our humanity. Rage diminishes it. Don't rehearse and dwell on offenses. Don't repeatedly remind people of their mistakes. Whenever possible, apologize and reconcile, even if it's not your fault. It gives the other person time to think and reciprocate.

Take Constructive Action

Taking constructive action as quickly as possible replaces the powerlessness and destructive power of problem anger with constructive power.

- Problem solve and get needed help (e.g., repair your computer or car).

- When angry, release the energy of fight or flight. If you are in a car, stop, get out, and walk around. If you are home, go for a walk, unload the dishwasher, clean, garden, exercise, etc.

- Learn skills: parenting, relationship enhancement, communication, and conflict resolution.

- Use requests to initiate, which are more effective than requests to stop (e.g., "Please clean up what you mess up," instead of "Stop leaving a mess.").

- Distract. After processing and learning from it, try to forget about it (i.e., think about other things, so as not to stew).

Walk the Peaceful Path

In interchanges with others, try to model calmness. Encourage others to talk, as you calmly listen. Try to show that you are trying to understand. Practice reassuring others. Help them save face. In many arguments, the real issue doesn't surface because the communication degenerates to attacks and trying to save face. Rather than criticizing the other person for coming home late ("You selfish and insensitive jerk!"), you might get to the heart of the issue by saying, "I'm disappointed because I didn't get to spend time with you last night."

Don't Drink Alcohol or Take Drugs

Avoid alcohol and drugs. You'll need your best thinking to practice complex anger skills. Likewise, don't drive when angry.

Have Patience and Persistence

If you have difficulty managing anger, it is not because you are deficient or bad. It is because you have not yet learned how.

I'm thinking of a young man in my anger class. He said that he had always felt like a bad person because he got so angry. He tried to bottle up his anger and it inevitably exploded. Listening to others in the class, he realized it was normal to get angry. As he learned ways to appropriately handle the anger, his anger diminished.

In your journey toward anger mastery, be prepared for tactical losses from time to time. These setbacks are common and won't negate your progress. If you persist, however, the long-term benefits will make your efforts well worthwhile.

Beware the Anger Myths

Myths about anger can interfere with your progress. The Anger Myths include the following:

Venting, or taking it out on others, decreases anger. This actually reinforces the neural networks associated with the anger response. Becoming angry affords practice in being angry, making us angrier people. Anger feeds anger.

Strong anger is necessary to change situations. Angry demands only appear to get the power we want. Often alternatives such as strong insistence, persistence, respect, and friendliness are more effective and bring results that are more long lasting. Do you like it when others treat you with contempt? Often strong anger breeds resentment and rebellion, and is transmitted transgenerationally.

If I don't get angry, I don't care. Anger is only one way to show that we care. Care can be shown with patient, disciplined, loving attention—as well as by firmness, giving of time, and sharing.

One who makes me mad is worthless and deserves my wrath. Dehumanizing others like this preserves one's anger. Humans are flawed and sometimes agonizingly slow to catch on, but not worthless.

Reducing anger means I think the offender isn't wrong. It only means you are learning ways to deal with offenses more coolly, effectively, and constructively.

The world is full of idiots and irritations. It is also full of beauty. The problem is not only the world's imperfections and provocations, but our chosen focus and reactions.

Men and women experience anger differently. Studies show that men and women get angry for the same reasons, as often, and with the same intensity. Behaviorally, however, men are more likely to manifest anger with physical or verbal assaults. Women are more likely to cry (which is more likely to help them get in touch with the underlying hurt).

Depression is anger turned inward. Depression is sadness, usually coupled with low self-esteem. However, depressed people often show higher levels of anger and anxiety. Anger expression is associated with any type of pain—including mental illness. Any type of mental illness that decreases the capacity for logical thought also increases the likelihood of anger and/or violence. Violent people are two to three times more likely to have a psychiatric illness such as depression.

Anger is a pure, basic emotion. Anger doesn't occur alone. Anger follows feelings such as fear, embarrassment, humiliation, shock, powerlessness, hurt pride, rejection, or pain. Ask: "What was I feeling first, before the anger?" This suggests the antidote to problem anger.

People make me mad. I can't control my anger. Remember that you usually control your anger when your boss corrects you or when a police officer gives you a ticket because you don't want to get fired or go to jail. It is true that the more one reinforces the habit of anger, the more difficult it is to control. However, new habits can be mastered and reinforced the more you practice them.

Drills

- Notice weaknesses, insecurities, or fears in another person; then hopes, strengths, and reasons to like that person.
- Replace anger, hostility, or malice with compassion (e.g., look at someone's face and try to sense their hurts).

Reflections

Violence is not strength, and compassion is not weakness.
(King Arthur in *Camelot*)

If you want *others* to be happy, practice compassion. If *you* want to be happy, practice compassion.
(Dalai Lama)

Man is born for mutual help, anger for mutual destruction.
(Seneca)

Hatred . . . is never positive. It has no benefit at all. It is always totally negative.
(Dalai Lama)

What do we live for if not to make life less difficult for each other?
(George Eliot)

Anger cannot be overcome by anger. If a person shows anger to you, and you respond with anger, the result is disastrous. In contrast, if you control anger and show opposite attitudes—compassion, tolerance, and patience—then not only do you yourself remain in peace, but the other's anger will gradually diminish.

(Dalai Lama, *A Policy of Kindness*)

Even our anger can be held with a heart of kindness.

(*Buddha's Little Instruction Book*)

I'd like to be an equal among equals; helping to lift, rather than competing; trying to contribute, not shine.

(Anonymous)

Suggested Activity

In your anger journal, ask, "Why am I getting angry?" Explore the feelings underneath the anger. Simply acknowledge and accept these feelings as part of being human.

PART II

Anger Management Skills

3

Cooling Down

*Nothing gives one person so much advantage over
another as to remain always cool and unruffled under all
circumstances.*

—Thomas Jefferson

Reducing Physical Arousal

The mind and the body are connected. One way to calm a sensitized nervous system, and thus increase the tendency to remain cool
under pressure, is to calm the body. Many people find the skills in
this chapter to be quite effective in their own right. These skills will
also help to prepare you for some of the more powerful skills discussed later in the book.

Anger triggers the stress response. When the brain senses a
threat, it initiates a chain of changes in the body. Neural and hormonal messages tell the body to prepare for fight or flight. In
response to these messages, the heart beats faster and more forcefully. Blood pressure and breathing rate increase. The levels of fats
and sugars in the blood increase. In the wisdom of the body, all of
these changes are adaptive in the short term. That is, they help to

provide the fuel and oxygen that the cells of the body require for the physical demands of fight or flight. The stress response (fight or flight) is designed to mobilize the body for physical action. This action expends the energy of the stress response, whereupon the body normally returns to the relaxed state. The stress hormones can even sharpen one's thinking in the short term.

In today's hectic, sedentary world, we have fewer physical outlets for the energy of stress. Moreover, before one's body can return to normal, new stressors often arise that keep the body aroused. It is when the arousal of stress is chronically elevated that problems occur. Stress hormones that remain elevated in the blood for long periods can become toxic to certain cells of the body. Elevated fats in the blood increase the risk of cardiovascular diseases. The immune system weakens, theoretically placing one at greater risk for infectious diseases and perhaps cancer. Moods slip and exhaustion is more likely. Another important negative outcome is that the nervous system becomes sensitized—the structure and function of the nerves change so that smaller irritations are now more likely to trigger a full-blown stress/anger response.

Anger is a form of stress that keeps the nervous system on alert. The sensitized nervous system then keeps the body on alert, or aroused.

An insidious, frequently overlooked physical change in chronic arousal is a shift in the way people breathe. When under stress, muscles around the abdomen, chest, throat, and jaw contract. This leads to rapid, shallow "chest breathing," or hyperventilation. Such breathing changes the chemistry of the blood, and makes the heart work harder. In one of the ironies of the body, hyperventilation also helps to keep the nervous system sensitized. Now a vicious cycle ensues. Chronic stress sensitizes the nervous system. A sensitized nervous system leads to hyperventilation. Hyperventilation keeps the nervous system sensitized.

Calm Breathing

One way to break this vicious cycle is to change the way we breathe. More precisely, we can return to the way we breathed as babies. Watch the way sleeping babies breathe—low, slowly, and deeply.

There is very little movement in the chest area. Rather, the abdomen slowly moves up and down with successive breaths.

Abdominal breathing is a very effective antidote to stress and anger. When the chest remains relatively still and quiet, respiration is essentially controlled by the diaphragm, a curved muscle below the lungs. When we inhale, the diaphragm contracts, creating a vacuum in the lungs that draws air in. When we exhale, the diaphragm relaxes. Abdominal breathing pulls air down into the deepest parts of the lungs, where air exchange is most efficient. Low and slow abdominal breathing is restful because skeletal muscles relax, and the heart and lungs do not need to work as hard.

Practice abdominal breathing lying down. This helps to relax the skeletal muscles that are not essential to breathing. Place one hand over the sternum, or breastbone, and the other hand over the navel. Notice which hand(s) move. If the upper hand is moving, this indicates inefficient chest breathing. Try to relax your throat, jaw, shoulders, chest, and abdomen, so that only your lower hand is moving. Imagine that your stomach is a balloon that fills with air when you inhale, and deflates when you exhale. Think of breathing gently into the hand that is over your navel. Let your abdomen rise softly into that hand, while your upper hand remains relatively still. The breaths are quiet and natural, one flowing smoothly into the other, with perhaps only slight pauses between exhalations and inhalations. Don't force your breathing to slow. However, you might notice that your breathing will become slower and more regular on its own accord. Practice this several times a day. Some people prefer to place a thick book, such as a phone book, over the navel. This helps them see the abdomen move, and actually strengthens the diaphragm. After a week's practice, consciously try to slow your rate to six to ten breaths per minute.

A few tips will help you to breathe more calmly throughout the day.

• Check your posture. Type As tend to stand in an attack posture. That is, they tighten their stomach and raise their chest and shoulders. This promotes hyperventilation. Try slouching down in a relaxed slump. Then imagine that you have a hook on the crown of your head. Imagine a string pulling your head straight up toward the ceiling, while your shoulders, stomach, and chest remain relaxed. Straightening the spine in this way while relaxing the abdomen disinhibits breathing. Keeping most of the skeletal muscles relaxed is also less fatiguing.

• Consciously relax the muscles in the face, since muscle tension tends to spread.

• Do not wear tight clothes, especially clothes that are tight around the waist.

• Consciously try to talk slower, permitting yourself to breathe normally. Talking so fast that one must gasp for air raises blood pressure.

Easy, Deep Breaths

Easy, deep breaths are simple and fast to learn, and are effective for almost all people who try them. When practiced frequently, they tend to calm the nervous system. Once the skill is solidified, easy, deep breaths can be used in stressful situations to quickly calm the aroused mind and body.

First, think of a calming word or phrase that will remind you to calm down. For instance, you might choose words such as *relax, peace, calm down, anger won't help*, or *I can handle this*.

Then, consciously breathe abdominally for a few moments. Remember to relax the face and all the muscles in the abdomen and upper body.

Now take two easy, deep breaths, saying your calming word or phrase as you breathe in and as you breathe out. Continue to relax your skeletal muscles, and only move your abdomen as you breathe. The breaths are still quiet and gentle, just a bit deeper than usual. So, as you inhale, you might say to yourself slowly, "Relax," letting the word spread out across the entire inhalation phase. As you exhale, you slowly repeat the same word. Or you might prefer a phrase such as "Calm down" on the inhalation, and a phrase such as "It'll be all right" on the exhalation.

Progressive Muscle Relaxation (PMR)

Progressive muscle relaxation (PMR) is the first form of structured relaxation developed in the West. Its originator, Dr. Edmund Jacobson, demonstrated that when people consciously relaxed their muscles, they became mentally calmer at the same time. Jacobson found, however, that simply trying to relax is only partially effective. One must paradoxically increase muscle tension for a while in order to help the brain to deeply relax the muscles. Thus, Jacobson developed a procedure to progressively tense the major muscle groups of the body, and then deeply relax those same muscle groups. As one progresses from one muscle group to another, the body becomes more and more relaxed (that is, muscle tension progressively decreases). Perhaps more importantly, the nervous system becomes more and more calm. In controlled research, PMR has been found to reduce blood pressure. It is also a very effective treatment for insomnia.[1]

PMR is a very active form of relaxation. It requires the expenditure of physical energy, and effectively distracts people from angry thoughts. It is effective for relaxing almost everyone who tries it. When anger management programs are short on time, this is the one form of structured relaxation that is most often taught. Thus, we taught this at the Pentagon, along with the breathing exercises described earlier.

Using this strategy, we progressively tense and then relax the major muscle groups of the body. You'll tense for about five to ten seconds, and then relax that same muscle group for at least that long. It is important to fully concentrate on how the states of tension and relaxation feel, and to notice the contrast between these states. PMR is not simply a very effective relaxation exercise; it is also a process of retraining the brain to distinguish between tension and relaxation. Many adults have become used to being chronically tense. As the brain regains the ability to deeply relax the muscles and then detect the first intimation of tension, you will then be able to use this information to catch yourself becoming tense or angry, and then consciously relax.

Progressive Muscle Relaxation Instructions

You can read this script through and then follow the summary. Alternatively, you might put the instructions on an audiotape and listen to them as you practice. You might also have someone read the instructions to you, or you might read them to another person (which is a good way to reinforce your own learning).

Prepare for this strategy by taking off glasses, contact lenses, and/or shoes, and loosening any tight clothing. Lie down in a comfortable place, with your arms at your sides. For comfort, you might wish to place pillows under your knees, the small of the back, and your head. (You can also do this in a seated position, with obvious adaptations of the instructions.) Try to stay alert and avoid sleeping as you practice this relaxation skill (unless, of course, you are practicing this in bed as an aid to sleep). Starting with the feet, we will progressively tense and then deeply relax the major muscle groups of the body. Remember to fully concentrate—first on the sensation of tension, and then on the contrast, the state of relaxation. Tense relatively hard, but always stop short of discomfort or cramps.

1. *To begin, please let your eyes close.* Notice the gentle, pleasant rhythm of your breathing—the cool, energizing air of the in-breath, and the relaxing release and sinking downward of the out-breath. Remembering your calming word or phrase, take two easy, deep abdominal breaths, saying your calming word or phrase slowly as you breathe in and again as you breathe out. Then return to the gentle rhythm of quiet, normal abdominal breathing. For a moment, notice what your body feels like. Notice any areas of tension in the body and release that tension.

2. *When I say* tense, *I'd like you to point both of your feet and toes at the same time, leaving the legs relaxed.* Notice the pulling sensation, or tension, in the calves and the bottoms of the feet. Form a clear mental picture of this tension. Now relax all at once. Feel the relaxation in those same areas. When muscles relax, they elongate, and blood flow through them increases. So you might feel warmth

or tingling in areas of your body that you relax. Just let your feet sink into the floor, completely relaxed.

3. *Next, pull your toes back toward your head.* Ready? Tense. Observe the tension in the muscles below the knee, along the outside of the shins. Now relax all at once and see and feel the difference as those muscles fully relax and warm up.

4. *Next, you'll tense the quadricep muscles on the front part of the leg above the knee by straightening your leg and locking your knees.* Leave your feet relaxed. Ready? Tense. Concentrate on the pulling in these muscles. See it clearly in your mind. And relax. Scan your quadriceps as you relax. Sense them loosening and warming, as though they are melting.

5. *Imagine now that you are lying on your back on a beach blanket.* The back of your heels are against the sand, and your toes are pointing toward the sky. Keeping your feet relaxed, imagine pressing the back of the heels into the sand. Ready? Tense. Feel and see the tension along the backs of the entire legs. Now relax as those muscles loosen and relax.

6. *A different set of muscles, those between the upper legs, are tensed when you squeeze your knees together.* Ready? Tense. Observe the tension. Then relax and observe the relaxation as you deeply relax, and keep relaxed, all the muscles in the legs as we progress upward. Just let the floor support your relaxed legs.

7. *Next you'll squeeze the buttocks, or seat muscles, together while contracting your pelvis muscles.* Let your stomach relax as you do this. Ready? Tense. Visualize the tension in these muscles. Then relax and observe what relaxation in those muscles is like—perhaps a pleasantly warm and heavy feeling.

8. *Next you'll tense your stomach muscles by imagining your stomach is a large ball and you want to squeeze it into a tiny ball.*

Ready? Tense. Shrink your stomach and pull it back toward the spine. Notice the tension there and how tensing these muscles interferes with breathing. Now relax. Let the abdomen warm up and loosen up, freeing your body to breathe in the least fatiguing way. Continue to breathe abdominally as you progress.

9. *Now leave your shoulders and buttocks down on the floor as you gently and slowly arch your back*. As you do, pull your chest up and toward your chin. You'll observe the tension in the back muscles along both sides of the spine. Now gently and slowly relax as your back sinks into the floor, feeling very warm and relaxed. Study that feeling. Notice where relaxation is experienced.

10. *Stabilize the lower back muscles by pressing the lower back against the floor*. Ready? Tense. Observe the tension, then relax and observe the relaxation.

11. *Prepare to press your shoulders downward, toward your feet, while you press your arms against the sides of your body*. Ready? Tense. Feel the tension in the chest, along the sides of the trunk, and along the back of the arms. You may not have been aware of how much tension can be carried in the chest or what that feels like. Relax, and feel those muscles loosen and warm. Realize that you can control and release the tension in your upper body once you are aware of it.

12. *Now, shrug your shoulders*. Ready? Tense. Pull them up toward your ears and feel the tension above the collarbones and between the shoulder blades, where many headaches originate. Now relax and study the contrast in those muscles.

13. *Place your palms down on the floor*. Pull your relaxed hands back at the wrists so that the knuckles move back toward your head. Observe the tension on the top of the forearms. Relax and study the contrast.

14. *Next, make tight fists and draw them back toward the shoulders as if pulling in the reins on a team of wild horses.* See the tension in the fists, forearms, and biceps. Relax and notice the feelings as those muscles go limp and loose. Just let your arms fall back beside your body, palms up. Heavy and limp and warm. Pause here to scan your body and notice how good it feels to give your muscles a break. Allow your entire body to remain relaxed as you move on.

15. *Let's learn how to relax the neck muscles, which typically carry much tension.* Right now, gradually, slowly turn your head to the right as if looking over your right shoulder. Take ten seconds or longer to rotate the neck. Feel the tension on the right side of the neck pulling your head around. The sensation on the left side is stretching, not tension. Hold the tension for a while to observe it. Then turn your head slowly back to the front and notice the difference as the muscles on the right side of your neck relax. Pause. Turn just as slowly to the left and feel the left side of your neck contract. Rotating back to the front, feel the left side relax.

16. *Now press the back of your head gently against the floor, while raising the chin toward the ceiling.* Do you notice the tension at the base of the skull, where the skull meets the neck? Much headache pain originates here, too. Study the tension. And relax. Allow those muscles to warm up and elongate. Relax the neck all around and let it remain relaxed.

17. *Lift your eyebrows up and furrow your brow.* Feel the tension along the forehead. Relax. Imagine a rubber band loosening.

18. *Wrinkle up your nose while you squeeze your eyes shut and your eyebrows together.* Observe the tension along the sides of the nose, and around and between the eyes. Now deeply relax those areas. Imagine pleasantly cool water washing over the eyes, relaxing them. Your eyelids are as light as a feather.

19. *Frown, pulling the corners of the mouth down as far as they'll go.* Feel the tension on the sides of the chin and neck. Relax. Feel the warm, deeply relaxing contrast.

20. *The jaw muscles are extremely powerful and can carry much tension. When I say* tense, *clench your jaw.* Ready? Tense. Grit your teeth and feel the tension from the angle of the jaw all the way up to the temples. Study the tension. Now relax and enjoy the contrast, realizing that you can control tension here, too. Relax the tongue and let the teeth part slightly.

21. *Make a wide smile.* Open the mouth wide. Ready? Tense. Grin from ear to ear and feel the muscles around the cheekbones contract. This really requires little effort. Now relax and let all the muscles of the face be soft and completely relaxed.

Allow a pleasant sense of relaxation to surround your body. Imagine that you are floating well supported on a favorite couch, bed, or raft—all your muscles pleasantly relaxed. When you are ready to end this session, count slowly to five, send energy to your limbs, stretch, sit up slowly, and move your limbs before standing slowly.

Practice this once or twice a day for two weeks or more. At first you might be more aware of aches or tension in your muscles. This tends to disappear with practice as those tense muscles get a break and your nerves desensitize. With practice, you'll notice that you can relax your muscles passively, by just reminding yourself to relax them. Some people use a reminder, such as a dot on their watch or a picture on the wall, as a cue to relax their muscles throughout the day.

Try to become increasingly aware of the first signs of tension and then cause those muscles to relax.

Relaxation Record

Keeping track of your practice and progress can be very motivating and revealing. Keep a Relaxation Record for several weeks using the form in Exhibit 3.1.

Exhibit 3.1 Relaxation Record

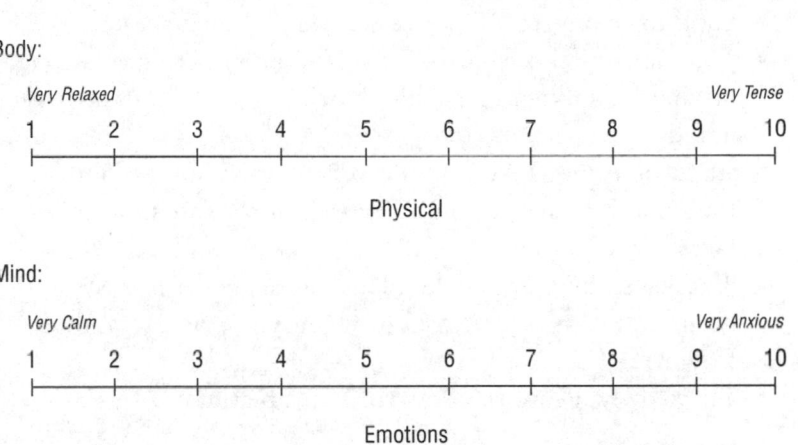

Body:

Very Relaxed									*Very Tense*
1	2	3	4	5	6	7	8	9	10

Physical

Mind:

Very Calm									*Very Anxious*
1	2	3	4	5	6	7	8	9	10

Emotions

Day/ Date	Time of Day	Length of Time	Physical		Mental/Emotional		Comments
			before	*after*	*before*	*after*	

Drills

- Look in the mirror. Remove scowls and grimaces.
- Consciously relax your body as you are walking, working, driving, or talking to people. Notice how this affects your mood.
- Stand in a line. Take easy, deep breaths. Look around for something interesting or beautiful to watch. Study faces.
- Practice smiling at people. (This causes fewer stress hormones to be secreted than when you grimace and frown.)
- Talk slowly. Pause to allow time to breathe.

Reflections

He who gives way to violent gestures will increase his rage.

(Darwin)

Conversely, he who talks slowly, smiles, and relaxes his muscles decreases his rage.

Suggested Activities

1. Practice taking two easy, deep breaths six times a day for at least three days—when you wake up, when you retire, before meals, and at other low-stress times. For the first day, try it lying down. On the second day, try it sitting down. On the third day, try it during slightly stressful times, such as when you are stopped at a traffic light. Record your progress on the Relaxation Record (see below).
2. Practice progressive muscle relaxation twice a day for at least two weeks. Record your progress on the Relaxation Record.

4

Calm Thinking

*Men are disturbed not by things, but the views which
they take of them.*

—Epictetus

MARGE AND JIM were talking by the watercooler about a project
they'd been working on. The boss brushed past them without giving his usual greeting. Jim thought, "Oh, no! He doesn't like our
work. I just don't get that guy! Nothing ever pleases him. I'm getting so sick of that idiot's arrogance. He thinks he's better than me."
Marge thought, "The boss seems so preoccupied lately. I know he's
under pressure from the front office, and having trouble at home."
Jim angrily stewed for the next hour. Marge felt concerned and a bit
upset, but was able to return to work with calm concentration. Same
event; different responses. What was the difference?

Cognitive therapy is a form of psychology that helps us understand how the thoughts we habitually choose lead to emotional disturbance. It helps us to identify those thoughts, challenge them, and
then replace them with cooler thoughts that enable us to react with
reasonable upset, rather than dysfunctional disturbance. Cognitive
therapy is a very well-researched approach that was originally devel
oped to treat depression. It has since been applied very effectively to

the treatment and prevention of anxiety, and now is a mainstay in the management of problem anger. The A-B-C model of cognitive therapy is straightforward:[1]

$$A \longrightarrow B \longrightarrow C$$

"**A**" stands for the Anger Trigger. "**B**" is the Belief (or automatic thoughts) that we tell ourselves about **A**. And "**C**" represents the emotional and physical Consequences of anger. Most people think that **A** is responsible for **C**. In reality, **B** has the greater influence. Hot thoughts lead to hot emotions, elevated physical arousal, and often poor functioning under pressure. Cooler thoughts result in less anger, less physical arousal, and a greater capacity to focus and concentrate on what we need to do when the world around us is in crisis. We may not always be able to control the outside world, but we each have the capacity to control ourselves.

Automatic Thoughts and Distortions

When anger triggers occur, *automatic thoughts* (ATs) run through our mind. Although we are each capable of thinking reasonably about these events, sometimes our automatic thoughts are *distorted*, or unreasonably negative. Distorted ATs occur so rapidly that we hardly notice them, let alone stop to question them. Yet these ATs profoundly affect our anger, our body's arousal, and our ability to function calmly.[2]

Distortions are simply thought habits that do not serve us very well. They are not a reflection of poor intelligence. They are simply picked up along the way—often from family, friends, or other life experiences—and thereafter not challenged. ATs are sometimes distorted because we are human and fallible, not inherently weak. When we learn the skills of identifying, logically challenging, and replacing these distorted ATs with more functional thoughts, anger levels fall dramatically.

The distortions that fuel excessive anger fall into only twelve categories. Learn them well. Identifying, rebutting, and replacing them are essential anger management skills that will also improve your over-all mental health and functioning. In your daily living, you will learn to frequently ask yourself: "Is this thought reasonable? Is it func-tional—that is, is it helping me? What if I thought in a different way?"

Before we begin to explore the common distortions, please con-sider this question: As human beings, what are our greatest fears? Death and public speaking aside, people usually mention events such as rejection, mistakes, failure to reach important goals, and criti-cism. Why? Such events can diminish feelings of being valued by others or our feelings of worth. If you understand this, then you will understand peoples' perfectionism ("If I'm perfect I won't be rejected"), failure rage ("It's awful to disappoint myself or to look bad"), and moral imperatives ("You shouldn't make me look so fool-ish because I need your respect"; "I must not tire or make mis-takes"). You will see them as fueled by fear and insecurity. This understanding leads to compassion for others (e.g., "That poor per-son has low self-esteem. I wonder if I can help."). It can also lead to compassion for oneself for having similar human insecurities. Para-doxically, acknowledging our insecurities and addressing them with compassion are first steps toward developing inner security.

The Distortions

1. *Irritation Fixation.* Here we focus on what is wrong or irri-tating. It's like having a mental camera that automatically zooms right in on anger hooks, blocking out the more pleasant aspects of the picture. For example:

- A father criticizes his son for an error in a baseball game, ignoring all the things that the son did well. That same father played a fine round of golf, but stewed for hours over the easy putt that he missed.
- Bill and Jasmine took a hundred-mile bike trip in Maine. Jasmine held on to the fact that one driver who passed them (out of hundreds) sat on his horn and shouted at them to get off the road. (By contrast, Bill thought, "That's just one driver in two thousand.")

- Carlos remembers with great irritation the time that his friend was late for an important appointment. He overlooks the fact that the friend is generally on time.
- Aaron still angrily remembers the one mistake in an otherwise stellar career that cost him a promotion. He thinks, "That one lousy error ruined my career."
- A father concentrates on his child's C and doesn't praise the As and Bs on the report card.

The problem with this narrow view is that it ignores the very aspects that make life satisfying and enjoyable.[3] And through conditioning and force of habit, we begin to find more and more reasons to be angry.

The antidote is to expand our focus—use a wider lens to see the whole picture. Ask: "What else could I notice? What *isn't* wrong? What's gone well? What is right or pleasant? What percentage of the time did I perform well? What's here to enjoy? Would I motivate others more by complimenting rather than criticizing? Would I motivate myself more with back pats rather than self-condemnation? Am I giving myself and others credit, when credit is due?" Notice that the suggestion is not to ignore the negative aspects, but to see *more* aspects. In short, we might ask, "What could I be grateful for if I were not taking such a critical posture?"

2. *Assuming.* There are two kinds of assumptions:

- *Mind Reading.* Here we assume that we know what others are thinking, without checking it out. For example, I once stopped at a gas station and asked the attendant for a rag to check the oil. He gruffly handed me one. I inquired, "You seem angry. Are you?" He said, "Oh, that last driver from New Jersey was so rude to me." He was angry, but it was not with me. Our first assumption is just one possibility among several to consider. Other examples and replacement thoughts are listed in Table 4.1.

Table 4.1 Replacing Mind Reading Assumptions

Mind Reading Assumptions	Replacement Thoughts
She thinks she's superior to me.	Perhaps. Or maybe she's keeping her distance because she's afraid.
You have an argument and assume that the other person doesn't respect you. "He thinks I'm stupid."	We just have different points of view. Maybe he's not thinking much about me at all. And if he does think I'm stupid, so what?
The service is slow and you think, "The waitress thinks I'm not important."	Maybe she's new or overwhelmed. Maybe the cook is slow.
The boss looks irritated. She is disappointed with my report.	I won't know that for sure unless I ask her. She might just be having a bad day.
She's deliberately trying to hurt me with her criticism. She takes pleasure in putting me down.	Maybe she cares about me, but is genuinely hurt by my behavior. Maybe she doesn't know how to be tactful. Maybe she wants to keep me from suffering by repeating that behavior. Maybe she's afraid of being misunderstood. Maybe she's having a bad day.
She didn't call. She's angry with me. She has some nerve!	Maybe there are other reasons for her not calling. I'd need to ask to be sure.
He's late because he doesn't respect me.	Perhaps lateness doesn't signify the same thing to him as it does to me. Maybe there are other reasons for his being late.
She doesn't like me.	I don't know that for sure.

Table 4.2 Replacing Fortune Telling Assumptions

Fortune Telling Assumptions	Replacement Thoughts
People who are different from me will hurt me.	Maybe not. If I reach out, they might turn out to be safe, perhaps even friends.
If I go to the party, I'll have a rotten time.	I might have a mediocre or somewhat enjoyable time. Maybe some aspects will be pleasant. I won't really know until I experiment.
If I try to talk about why I'm angry, I'll lose control and look like an idiot.	If I am earnest and try to be reasonable, perhaps I'll do a reasonably good job. Perhaps it will help understanding to grow and the relationship to improve.
If I express my anger, I'll explode. I'll become violent and beat my kids, just like Dad did to me.	I can verbalize feelings. That's different from acting on them. In fact, only a minority of adults who were abused as children abuse their own children.

- *Fortune Telling.* Here we pessimistically predict a negative outcome without testing the evidence. Table 4.2 lists examples of such assumptions and possible replacement thoughts.

  Fortune telling often starts with a fear focus—"It *might* happen. After all, it's happened before. Or, it could happen for the first time."—and subtly shifts to a "It will *undoubtedly* happen," which further arouses. To challenge this distortion, we need to think more tentatively and openly, like a scientist. "Certainly bad things might happen, but what's the probability or odds of this happening?" Other antidotes include thinking, "Why might this negative *not* happen? Sometimes good things happen."

3. *Catastrophizing* is making things much worse than they actually are. We assume that something is so horrible, dreadful, disas-

Table 4.3 Replacing Catastrophizing

Catastrophizing	Replacement Thoughts
This is outrageous and intolerable. I can't stand it when things don't go the way I want!	It's inconvenient and I don't like it, but I *can* stand it.
It's awful if others disrespect me. It's horrible to look weak in front of others.	That's disappointing, but is it really that big of a deal in the grand scheme of things? Should I really let someone else's opinion disturb my peace of mind?
I hate to be disrespected.	I don't have to take this too seriously. Twenty years from now, will this seem that important? Five years from now? How much will I really care about this when I die?
It's awful to feel helpless and out of control.	That's okay. That's life. Everyone feels this way sometimes. It's normal.
His behaviors are interfering with my career goals, material success, and reputation. How awful!	This is understandably annoying. but I don't have to let him disturb my peace of mind. In a way, I can thank that person for saving me from the pitfalls of fame, greed, bondage to material wealth, having too many things to manage, having more demands on my time, and being valued for my wealth. Maybe this isn't all bad.

trous, or awful that we can't stand it. In exaggerating the badness or danger of the situation, we also magnify our arousal and create a feeling of helplessness. Table 4.3 lists examples of catastrophizing, along with suggested replacement thoughts.

There is often an unrecognized element of fear in catastrophizing. It might start with a *What if* . . . ("What if this awful thing happens! What if I screw up again! What if I can't change this situation! What if I'm overwhelmed and can't cope!"). "What ifs" keep the focus on the worst possible fear, so we remain aroused, while distracting us from what we can resolutely do to maximize the possibility of a good outcome.

The goal in dealing with catastrophizing is to stay calm, neither under- nor overestimating the threat, so that we can reasonably and appropriately select the best strategy. The many rebuttals to this pervasive distortion may be summarized as follows:

- Ask, "So what? How likely is this to do me in? Will the world really end?"
- Think, "It's not so bad. This is inconvenient, not a catastrophe."
- Think, "Okay, let's assume the worst is really happening or will happen. What will I *do* then?" There is something calming about fully facing the worst, accepting that it could happen or is happening, and then determining what you would or can do to improve it. Turn a *What if* . . . into an *If then* . . . ("If such and such happens, then I'll do such and such to make the best of the situation and salvage what I can.") For example, "If I were unable to fully recover from a mistake and were to lose my job, I'd grieve for a while; perhaps I'd retool, seek a new job, and enjoy life." Remind yourself that the negative may never happen, but if it does you'll make the most of it. Instead of "What if this negative happens?", ask "What if it doesn't?"
- To realize that there are many coping options, ask what others have done in similar situations. If, despite your best efforts, you can't change a negative situation, you might think, "This is the reality. Even though I don't like it, I accept it."

4. *All-or-Nothing Thinking.* Here we think in extremes that create arousal and often diminish self-esteem or one's opinion of others. Think of a pole vaulter who sets the bar very high and considers himself a loser for not making it over. There is no middle ground and no partial credit in this distortion. Examples of how to replace all-or-nothing thinking are presented in Table 4.4.

Notice that most humans operate in the middle ground much of the time. No one excels in all things at all times. Falling short of perfection makes humans fallible, not worthless. All you can do is your best. If you are already committed to doing your best, then

Table 4.4 Replacing All-or-Nothing Thinking

All-or-Nothing Thinking	Replacement Thoughts
Either I'm number 1, or I'm a loser. If I'm not superior, I'm inferior, I'm on top or I'm a flop.	This kind of thinking will drive me to compete constantly with others and myself, rather than living peacefully. Half of all brain surgeons are below average. Remembering this, I can do my personal best and give myself credit when I do, even if I fall short of perfection.
If I can't get my way, I am weak, helpless, out of control, or powerless.	I certainly can't get my way all the time, but that makes me human, not powerless. It's normal to sometimes be in situations where I don't have much control. That's life.
If I give in or compromise, I'm weak.	To bend is to be flexible and considerate of others, not weak.
If I'm not totally accepted, loved, or respected, I am totally disrespected or rejected.	I'd like to be generally well regarded, but it's silly to expect to be worshiped, since I am not perfect.
Only one of us can be right. Either one is right or one is wrong.	Such extremes rarely exist. Usually there is some validity to both sides of an argument.
You're with me or you're against me; friend or foe.	It's foolish to demand that someone agree with me on everything, since people will always have their own views of things. An honest disagreement doesn't necessarily mean someone is my enemy or doesn't appreciate me. Not everyone is out to get me. Some people might be against me, some will be friendly, and most will be indifferent.
They messed up. They're completely worthless and incompetent.	The fact that their *behavior* fell short of perfection doesn't mean they are worthless and incompetent overall.
If I make a mistake, I am a complete failure.	A mistake means I am human and fallible. I'm not a failure if I am trying my best.
I either will bottle up my anger or I will explode uncontrollably.	Perhaps I can find a middle ground, a way to express my anger constructively.

worrying or condemning yourself adds nothing to your performance. Worrying or condemning saps motivation and robs the joy of living in the moment. Rating your performance on a scale of 1 to 10 helps correct this distortion. For example, "I performed at about 80 percent today." (Notice, we rate *behavior*, not people, who are too complex to rate.) Also, redefine success as trying your best and progressing, not reaching perfection.

When applied to others, extreme thinking damages relationships. We will be very disappointed and angry if we expect perfection of others. Or we might avoid basically good people who are not 100 percent trustworthy but who are trying and improving. People are not all good or all bad, but are a combination of bad and good attributes, at varying degrees of development. It takes time to build trust and it can be earned and given in varying degrees. If we are willing to patiently walk in the middle ground, we might make better judgments about people and be disappointed less often.

In addition, extreme thinking might apply to the way we view the world and remember our experiences ("My dream vacation was ruined by that rude service"). There is a tendency to forget that some aspects were good and some were bad. That's the way life is, generally. To remember this lessens upset at the parts that are not yet going well.

Finally, extreme thinking includes the view that I am either strong or I am emotional. The middle ground might be, "I can be strong *and* have feelings. Having genuine feelings makes me human, not weak. Shedding a tear does not mean that I will become a complete basket case. *The constructive expression of feelings—hurt, sadness, fear—will let me bend without breaking.*"

5. *Shoulds (musts/oughts)* are rigid demands we make of ourselves, others, or the world. These demands insist that the world be somehow different than it is. The unspoken assumption is that the consequences are dire if the demand is not met. We are impressed at how frequently shoulds are found when anger is high. It is clear how this distortion keeps arousal high.

"Shoulding" on Self

- "I should have done better. I shouldn't have made that mistake."

- "I must be strong. I ought to be number one."
- "I must no longer make mistakes, since mistakes caused me pain in the past."
- "I shouldn't be afraid, tired, imperfect, etc."
- "I must not lose control."
- "I must be right."
- "I shouldn't be feeling so angry."

As with anger, shoulds attempt to protect the self from being diminished. Since we'll always perform less than perfectly, however, shoulds usually punish more than they protect. How do you feel when you tell yourself you should have been perfect when you weren't? Demanding a more favorable outcome when the unfavorable outcome has already occurred is counterproductive, and only makes us angrier. Perfectionistic demands for future performance only *seem* to motivate us. Research has shown, however, that aiming for a very good job actually improves performance better than grimly expecting perfection.

Preferential and intentional, rather than demanding, thinking can motivate without the anger. For example: "I prefer to stay calm. I want to be less angry because I choose to (i.e., because I see that it is in my best interest or the best interest of others), not because someone is telling me I should." "I'd like to be right, but it's not a dire necessity." "I probably would have done better if I'd . . . . Next time I'm going to try that."

Table 4.5 provides examples of "shoulding on others" thoughts, and then replacement thoughts.

"Shoulding" on the World

- "Bad things shouldn't happen to good people. I shouldn't have to suffer."
- "It's not fair. It should not have happened to me. Only good things should happen."

All "should" distortions share the fact that we create unrealistic expectations. We create levels that are too high and then expect the world to comply. It is okay to shoot high—to have strongly held beliefs about what will make the world a better place—as long as we are not surprised when others disagree, or when we fall short of our

Table 4.5 Replacing "Shoulds"

"Shoulding" on Others	Replacement Thoughts
You shouldn't be that way. You should know better.	One of the few reasonable shoulds is that people should be just the way they are, given their flawed upbringing, understanding, worldview, and ability to live up to their ideals. If people *really* knew better—that is, they knew how to be better, were capable of doing so, and realized that this would make them happier—wouldn't they be better?[4]
He must behave well. He must do it my way—now.	Why must he? People have free choice to behave poorly. They don't have to do anything I think is right. The world hasn't ended because people behave badly, although the world is certainly a nicer place when they don't. I'd prefer that he behave well.
That driver should pull over when I flash my lights. He should be banned from the road.	He probably doesn't share my opinion. Why should that get my goat?
Others shouldn't disrespect me.	Why not? They do it to others. Why should I be protected? Lots of people don't respect or treat themselves well. Is it reasonable to expect them to treat me better than they treat themselves? Why should this make me go postal?
You must not make me look bad. I must avenge that offense.	Everyone looks bad from time to time. So what? Usually the person who looks most foolish is the person who declares World War III for every minor offense.
He must not get away with that. I must correct injustice.	Why must I? Maybe the world won't end if I don't obsess about the trivial errors of others. In fact, my rigid insistence on fixing everyone might only needlessly put me in danger. Maybe I could let the police take care of the big offenses.
My authority must not be questioned.	Why not? It's not so bad, especially if it's respectfully done.

"Shoulding" on Others	Replacement Thoughts
Why can't you see things my way?	Often this means, "You shouldn't be so stupid. You should see things my way." Once I realize that different views are inevitable, I'll become more accepting and less angry.
I must keep my kids in line at all times. I must not allow them to mess up—ever.	No parents ever had perfect kids, no matter how demanding they were. If I kindly and gently support, set limits, lead by example, and allow them to be fallible, they'll probably turn out to be decent human beings.

hopes. Remember, a powerful antidote for a should is a *would* or a *could*. Woulds and coulds preserve ideals but in a gentler, more flexible way that accepts the world as it is. For example:

- "It *would* be nice to be less distressed during a crisis and perform more coolly. I wonder how I *could* do this."
- "It *would* be nice to see eye to eye, but people have separate realities. In the meantime, I wonder what I *could* be trying."
- "It *would* be nice if things were better. But I accept that . . .

  - people will always be fallible, never perfect."
  - life will always be unfair and things will happen that we don't always deserve."
  - no one can ever achieve total control of events."

- "I won't make myself crazy by insisting things be perfect right now. I'll just aim to do a very good job and expect I'll probably improve with experience."

Also ask, "Why should I? Where is this should written?" For example, is it written somewhere that humans should be perfect when they try a difficult task for the first time? Or the hundredth time?

A final antidote is to see what happens when you don't do the thing you think you must and realize that the world does not end (e.g., "If I allow myself to be vulnerable, I might learn that people like me better." "If I allow my children to make some mistakes they might learn some valuable lessons. This is not a combat zone, after all.").

Entitlement is a special form of should that says, "I am owed happiness, what I want, respect, wealth, etc." Nothing is promised. You might consider giving up entitlements, and replacing those expectations with hopes ("I would wish for . . .") and gratitude for what you do have.

6. *Feelings passing as facts* is thinking that your feelings represent reality. Often angry people feel so strongly that their anger is justified that they assume that it really is. Feelings of indignation then fan the flame of anger. Interestingly, criminals, gang members, spousal abusers, and aggressive road ragers also typically feel that their anger is justified—usually by past or present circumstances. The cooler outside observer would often disagree. So the antidote to this distortion is to become a cool "outside observer," realizing that when we are under stress our thoughts are not always reasonable or accurate. Other examples can be found in Table 4.6.

The goal is to treat feelings as a beloved, valued, trusted, but fallible friend. Pay attention to them and respect them, but allow that they can be wrong at times. Feelings can be colored by fatigue, pain, stress, or habitual attitudes. Ask yourself, "Is this reality or just a feeling?" If after calm analysis your anger does still seem justified, remember that you can be firm, resolute, and in control of your reactions—without hatred or bitterness. We think of the allied troops in the Gulf War. As a rule, they felt their cause was just, and they pursued it in a professional manner—capably, efficiently, and without bloodthirst or hatred.

7. *Overgeneralizing* is deciding that your negative experience applies to all situations. For example:

- "People always let you down. They always take advantage of you."

Table 4.6 Replacing "Feelings Passing as Facts"

Feelings Passing as Facts	Replacement Thoughts
I feel so strongly negative toward him. I must be justified.	This might just be a result of my hostile lens on people.
I feel so right.	Maybe I'm biased—missing some facts or a different perspective.
I feel like I'm allowing myself to be controlled by giving in.	I'm helping to build a better relationship. Compromising is not necessarily giving in.
I feel helpless, powerless, out of control.	I'm not really. I have options. (See constructive power meditation, page 121.)

- "All men want only one thing."
- "Everything in life is so unfair."
- "All of those people (whites, blacks, Jews, Christians, etc.) are like that."
- "Nobody ever listens to me."
- "My whole life stinks."
- "Things always go wrong. It never fails."
- "You never do what you say you will."
- "I always get in the slow lane."
- "I can't do anything right. I never do things right. I always let people down."

Words such as *always, never, everyone, nobody, all,* or *none* indicate overgeneralizations. The opposite of these words is *some* ("*Some*times I do pretty well"; "*Some* people are responsible *some*times"; "*Some* things turn out well."). Ask if a negative event could be an exception to the rule. Maybe the world isn't always like this.

Some people overgeneralize in the positive direction ("All the world is good and safe"; "All people are good."). When an irresponsible act occurs, they become embittered and disappointed. Again, the word *some* helps. For example, Hillary was raised by a decent, loving father. She assumed that all men are trustworthy. She was shocked when her boyfriend raped her. She learned to view reality on a continuum. Between the extremes of *men are totally trustworthy* and *men are untrustworthy,* she viewed a new middle ground: *Some men are generally trustworthy and some are generally untrustworthy.* She accepted responsibility to evaluate each individual separately.

8. *Abusive Labeling.* Here you give yourself or another person a label, or name, as though a single word could describe a complex person completely. For example, to say, "I am an idiot," means that I am *always* and *in every way* an idiot. Obviously, this isn't fair or true. Individuals often acquire the habit of internalizing critical comments as children, then continue to berate themselves when they reach adulthood. Berating oneself is of no use whatsoever. If you condemn yourself as stupid and unworthy, how can you see yourself in the future acting wisely and worthily? The antidote is to rate behavior, but not people. Thus, "I performed at about 65 percent today," rather than "I'm a loser."

Notice that labels can be levied at other people as well, which is common in anger reactions. To reduce another human being to an "always-and-in-every-way" label is just as inaccurate and unfair as doing it to yourself, even if it feels justified. To call someone incompetent or worthless to the core is unreasonable, because each person does something reasonably well (e.g., even a criminal can be an effective organizer; even someone who lies is sometimes honest). Rather than labeling someone, we might rate the behavior as undesirable. Thus, "That person's driving is poor today," is likely to induce less anger than a label of "worthless loser." People are fallible and are moved by disturbance, faulty logic, inattention, upbringing, and lack of preparation or skill—but humans are not worthless. Do you think that someone you know is inept? You might ask, "Is he always inept?" If not, you might release the label and replace it with an evaluation of his present behavior. If you conclude that the person is in fact always and in every way inept, you might ask, "Is he inept on purpose?" If the answer is yes, then ask, "Why should I let that bother me? The poor person must already be suffering from his choice." If the person is not intentionally inept, but is imperfect, troubled, or distracted—just like all of us at times—then you can let him off the hook.

9. *Personalizing* is seeing yourself as more responsible or involved than you really are. Table 4.7 illustrates ways in which we personalize events in angry ways and offers replacement thoughts.

10. *Blaming* places too much responsibility for your problems on something outside of yourself. For example, in spousal abuse classes for Marine drill instructors, one of the first steps is to challenge the distortion "My wife makes me angry." Nobody makes another person angry. We are responsible for our own anger. Other examples:

- "My ex treated me so miserably. He has ruined my life and my self-esteem."
- "I've been the victim. This justifies my anger and my behavior."
- "I'm angry because of _____ (my crummy childhood, Vietnam, the doctor's incompetence, etc.)."
- "I'm going down the tubes because I lost your love."

The problem with blaming, much like catastrophizing, is that it leads us to feel like helpless victims who are unable to control our own anger. Blaming keeps us stuck in the past problem, powerless since the past is unchangeable. It maintains anger by shifting responsibility for our present well-being away to someone or something else. In shifting the blame to others, we feel less vulnerable, but nothing really changes. The antidote to blaming is to acknowledge outside influences, but to take responsibility for your own welfare. "Okay, I see how these things have influenced my development and/or challenge me. Now I commit to get back on track and move

Table 4.7 Replacing Personalizing

Personalizing	Replacement Thoughts
That guy just cut me off! He's out for me.	His driving certainly is bad, but it's safe to say that it wasn't a personal attack since he doesn't even know me. Maybe he hates the world, not me. Maybe he is neutral to me or completely oblivious to me. Perhaps it wasn't even deliberate.
He dissed me. I'm personally offended.	It's really not personal. His hot buttons were in place long before this happened. Maybe I'm not the central character in his play. His offensive actions have personal meaning only if I give them meaning.
He's judging me negatively.	Maybe he's thinking about his own problems. Maybe he's mad because he had an argument with his wife. And if he doesn't think well of me, so what? What's the big deal?
Why did this happen to me? Why was I singled out?	The world is not for or against us. Both bad and good things happen to people.
I failed this test. What's wrong with me?	Simple. I'm imperfect. This was a difficult test, and I was stressed and tired when I took it. Instead of condemning myself, next time I'll prepare better and get more rest.
My kids are trying to goad me.	Maybe they don't know how to meet their needs.
If I hadn't nagged my son, he wouldn't have gotten drunk and gotten in that accident.	Influence is different from a cause. I'm not responsible for another person's choices.

on." For present hooks we might think, "Nothing makes me do any-thing—I now choose how I respond. I can choose to keep my peace." *Also, remember that nothing outside of yourself can make you feel diminished without your consent. You can be strong and secure inside so that someone outside can't really hurt you in a lasting way.* Ask yourself, "What's my best course of action?"

11. *Unfavorable Comparisons.* Here you magnify another's strengths and your weaknesses, while minimizing the other's faults and your strengths. So by comparison, you feel inadequate or inferior. Do you ever do this? It can be quite discouraging. Or it can lead to jealousy, anger, and the need to prove you are better than the other person. There is a destructive kind of competition wherein people are constantly trying to prove to other people (or themselves) that they measure up to others. To compensate for feeling vulnerable, we might put others down so that we look better by comparison. A way to challenge this distortion is to ask, "Why must I compare? Why can't I just appreciate that each person has unique strengths and weaknesses? Another's contributions are not necessarily better, just different." Or, you might think, "Okay, so I'm less powerful and effective than John in this area. Why is that so horrible? All I can do is my personal best." As a rule, you'll function better and with less stress when you focus on doing your personal best, not on comparisons.

12. *Regrets.* In looking back, we think, "If only I hadn't . . . (performed so poorly, been so angry, said what I did)." Beyond a period of introspection where mistakes are acknowledged, amends are made, and courses are corrected, regrets are unproductive because we can't go back and change the past. Chronic regrets keep us from accepting ourselves despite our inevitable imperfections. We might beat ourselves, thinking, "I deserve to be punished for that." This kind of pain can lead to more anger. What we actually deserve is the opportunity to try again, improve, and learn from the mistakes. We can think, "I've learned from mistakes in the past and I can do so again. That was then and this is now."

Notice that we are not suggesting that one brush off guilt. Rather, we can compassionately acknowledge the mistake. Instead of condemning ourselves, we can consider if the mistake was deliberate. If so, we might notice if it was made under duress, at a time when needed skills for handling intense feelings were lacking. Were there influences outside of your control that made this situation difficult? We can do all that is possible to restore the damage or apologize, learn ways to prevent a recurrence of the mistake, resolve to improve, and then move on without the weight of regrets.

It is a natural human tendency to feel guilt when we hurt another person or behave poorly. If we can calmly examine the guilt, we can grow and improve. Then guilt has done its work, and can be released.

A Final Word on Distortions

We noted that the use of distortions does not reflect intelligence, only dysfunctional, unchallenged habits. Distortions cannot only lead to anger, but physical illness as well. I once attended a lecture by noted hostility researcher Margaret Chesney with a Pentagon colleague. Dr. Chesney is an extremely congenial woman, and her lecture was very factual. Following the lecture linking hostility to heart disease, a man who was sitting in front of me raised his hand during the question period. With pursed lips, a forced smile, and jiggling foot, he leaned forward and said (see if you can notice the thought errors), "You make it sound like it's a sin for me to be angry. Some people deserve it. I have no choice. Otherwise I'll be a doormat." Do you see the distortions in his statements? He started with an accusatory statement, "You make it sound . . . " (Angry people frequently start their statements with "you," which tends to put people on the defensive.) "Like a sin for me to be angry" is a mind read and personalizing. "Some people deserve to be punished" overlooks the point that hostile people are already hurting and suffering for their choices. "I have no choice" misses the point that we always have a choice on whether to become angry or not. Becoming "a doormat" if one does not retaliate with anger is an all-or-nothing distortion.

The second part of the story is even more interesting to me. My colleague, a psychologist, leaned over and said, "He's a brilliant researcher. He's already had his first heart attack. Look at his wife." I had not previously noticed the woman sitting next to him. Her

Turn questions into statements when you identify your self-talk. For example, asking "Why can't I do this?" keeps us aroused and provides no resolution. Changed to the statements "I can't do this—I'm stupid" or "This shouldn't be so hard," the Abusive Labeling and Should distortions become obvious. We can then replace these distortions with a thought such as, "It's difficult because I don't know how yet."

"Why" questions are intellectual. The intellectual response is straightforward: "I am suffering because I haven't learned how not to yet." However, the real issue is the emotional frustration. It is better to directly state, "I am feeling so frustrated with this pain." Then take steps to soothe yourself as you learn additional skills.

body language was telling. She had her legs crossed and was turned away from him, as if to get as far away from him as possible. My colleague said, "She's seeing me for help to deal with her Type A husband." We've often wondered if intelligence is really useful if it is not used to improve health, happiness, and relationships.

The Daily Thought Record

Now that you know about distortions, the next step is to use them to help you. When stressed or angry, thoughts and feelings can swirl in our minds and seem overwhelming. Putting them down on paper helps us sort it all out and see things more clearly. One way to do this is through the Daily Thought Record[5] (Exhibit 4.1), which takes about fifteen to twenty minutes to complete. It is a good thing to do immediately after you notice yourself feeling upset; or you may approach the exercise later when you have calmed down. (See Exhibit 4.2 for an example of a completed Daily Thought Record.)

Each day for two weeks, select an upsetting event and do a Daily Thought Record. You might start with a specific hook that you encountered recently and progress to past or future hooks.

Remember, work out your thoughts on paper. It is too complex to do it in your head. Be patient with yourself as you learn how to do this. It usually takes a few weeks to become good at this skill.

Exhibit 4.1 The Daily Thought Record

Step 1: The Facts

At the top, briefly describe an upsetting event from the past, present, or future and the resulting feelings (such as anger, frustration, sadness). Rate the intensity of these feelings on a scale of 1 to 10, with 10 meaning extremely unpleasant. Remember, getting in touch with disturbing feelings is a way to stop them from controlling us.

Step 2: Analysis of Your Thoughts

In the left column of the Analysis section, list your Automatic Thoughts (ATs) separately. Then rate how much you believe each one. A 10 means it's completely believable.

In the middle column, identify the distortions. (Some ATs might be reasonable.)

In the right column, try to respond, or talk back, to each distorted AT. Realize that your first AT is only one of several possible choices. Try to imagine what you would say to a friend who said what you did, or try to imagine yourself on a good day saying something more reasonable. Ask yourself, "What is the evidence for the reasonable response?" Then rate how much you believe each response.

Step 3: Results

After all this, go back to the left column and rerate your ATs. Then at the top rerate the intensity of your emotions. Even a slight drop in your upset feelings is significant. With this process, upsetting events will still probably be upsetting, just not as intense or disturbing.

Date: _____

Daily Thought Record

The Facts

Event	Impact of Event	Intensity
(Describe the event that "made you" feel bad/unpleasant.)	*(Describe the emotions you felt.)*	*(Rate the intensity of these emotions from 1–10.)*

Analysis of Your Thoughts

Automatic Thoughts (ATs)		Distortions	Reasonable Responses	
(Describe the Automatic Thoughts or Self-Talk. Then rate how believable each is from 1-10.)	*Ratings*	*(Find and label the distortions.)*	*(Talk back! Change the distortions to more reasonable thoughts. Rate how much you believe each from 1–10.)*	*Ratings*

Results

Based upon your Thought Analysis, rerate how much you believe your initial responses.
Then rerate the intensity of your emotions.

Exhibit 4.2 The Daily Thought Record—A Completed Sample

This is an example of a Daily Thought Record. Mike was a strapping Marine officer who looked like John Wayne. His biggest hook was that three hundred people jumped when he gave an order at work, but his teenage son used his spotless truck without cleaning it afterward. After he completed the Daily Thought Record below, he still wanted to have his truck returned clean, and he was able to talk the situation over calmly and effectively with his son—without disturbed anger.

Date: June 10

Daily Thought Record

The Facts

Event	Impact of Event	Intensity
(Describe the event that "made you" feel bad/unpleasant.)	(Describe the emotions you felt.)	(Rate the intensity of these emotions from 1–10.)
Truck is a mess after my son uses it for his date.	Anger Disappointment	$9 \to 5$ $8 \to 6$

Analysis of Your Thoughts

Automatic Thoughts (ATs)		Distortions	Reasonable Responses	
(Describe the Automatic Thoughts or Self-Talk. Then rate how believable each is from 1-10.)		(Find and label the distortions.)	(Talk back! Change the distortions to more reasonable thoughts. Rate how much you believe each from 1–10.)	
	Ratings			Ratings
He's a slob.	$7 \to 4$	Label	Actually, he is very neat in matters that are important to him.	9
He should know better.	$9 \to 6$	Should	Just because I've taught him to be neat and orderly doesn't mean that he sees the value of keeping my truck spotless. I suppose if he really thought that cleaning it up would make him successful and happy, then he *would* clean it up.	8
This disobedience is awful.	$9 \to 7$	Catastrophizing	This is disappointing and frustrating, but pretty normal for teenagers. This isn't combat, or a life-or-death situation. There's time to calmly come up with a solution.	7
He doesn't respect me.	$7 \to 3$	Mind Reading	This is probably less about respect and more about the fact that he has other priorities.	7
He'll get fired from his job because he doesn't follow instructions.	$8 \to 6$	Fortune Telling	He's generally responsible and will probably complete assigned tasks that he considers important.	8

Getting to the Most Distressing Ideas: The Question-and-Answer Technique

So far you have learned to use the Daily Thought Record to identify and replace distorted ATs. While replacing distorted ATs can greatly reduce distressing emotions, uprooting *core beliefs* provides even greater relief.[6] Core beliefs are deeply held beliefs that lead to many present distortions. Because they are usually learned early in life, they are rarely challenged. We discover core beliefs by starting with an AT and using the question-and-answer technique. In this approach, you take an AT and keep asking the following questions until you reach the core belief:

Assuming that the AT is true:

* What does that mean to me?
* Why is that so bad?

For example, Marianne was a bright and popular graduate student. Her biggest hook was that her husband, a lawyer, ignored her when he was reading the paper. In response, she felt angry and resentful, and then guilty and silly for feeling angry. She easily rebutted her labeling ("He's insensitive") and overgeneralizing ("He always does this"). The AT that still seemed upsetting was "He thinks my opinions are insignificant." How she decided to apply the question-and-answer technique to this AT is illustrated in Exhibit 4.3.

In reaching this core belief, we did not pause to challenge the ideas. Now let's go back and look for distortions along the way, responding reasonably at each step. Exhibit 4.4 illustrates the entire process, using the three columns of the Daily Thought Record. (In this model, Q represents *Question*, which need not be written down.)

Core beliefs usually relate to some condition that we consider important for our happiness, such as being lovable or in control or powerful (this one tends to be more important for men).

Exhibit 4.3 The Question-and-Answer Technique to Uncover the Core Belief—A Sample

Automatic thought:	He thinks my opinion is insignificant.
Question:	What does that mean to me?
Answer:	Maybe what I'm saying *is* insignificant.
Question:	And what does that mean?
Answer:	I'm not intelligent.
Question:	And what does that mean?
Answer:	I'm not respected.
Question:	What does that mean? Why is that so bad? What does that say about you?
Answer:	I'm unlovable.
Question:	What does that mean? Why is that so bad?
Answer:	I can't be happy without his love. (= CORE BELIEF!)

Some Common Core Beliefs

Table 4.8 lists a number of core beliefs common to anger and their more reasonable alternatives. As a drill, cover up the alternatives and see how you would respond to each core belief. There are no perfect or "right" answers. What matters is that the response works for you.

For a week, use the question-and-answer technique once a day to determine your core beliefs. Use previously completed Daily Thought Records, or a newly completed Daily Thought Record.

Exhibit 4.4 Challenging Distortions

Automatic Thoughts (ATs)	Distortions	Reasonable Responses
He thinks my opinion is insignificant.	Mind Reading	Most of the time he enjoys hearing my ideas.
Q		
Maybe what I am saying *is* insignificant.	All-or-Nothing	I don't always have to be saying something brilliant.
Q		
I'm not intelligent.	All-or-Nothing	How silly. I'm certainly intelligent and show it in various ways.
Q		
I'm not respected.	Feelings Passing as Facts	He just likes to have a few minutes of quietude after work.
Q		
I'm unlovable.	Label	I suppose no one is totally lovable at every moment. But I certainly feel that I am generally lovable. And I don't need to let my value fluctuate according to someone else's reaction to me.
Q		
I can't be happy without his love. (Core Belief)	Fortune Telling	I certainly hope to always have his love. Should I lose that for any reason, I am smart enough to figure out ways to still be happy.

Rational Emotive Imagery

Rational emotive imagery, developed by the psychologist Albert Ellis, is a very effective way to reinforce the skills of cognitive therapy. Recalling the A-B-C model discussed earlier in this chapter (see page 68), imagine a hook, the self-talk, and the resulting feelings related to one of your hooks. Get a good mental picture of all of these.

Table 4.8 Common Core Beliefs and Alternatives

Core Beliefs	Alternatives
My worth is determined by winning, by coming out on top. If I lose or give in, my worth is diminished.	Human worth is too vast to be so narrowly defined. I don't equate my worth to winning.
I can't walk away from a fight.	Choosing to avoid confrontation is a strength when confrontation is pointless.
All people that I consider significant must love me.	It would be nice, but not a dire necessity.
It shows weakness to apologize or admit I'm wrong.	It shows wisdom and courage.
I must get angry to be respected.	Respect is earned by dependability, not anger.
My worth is a function of how others treat me, or what they think of me.	The way people think of you and treat you are more likely to be reflections of their opinions of themselves.
Only she can meet my needs; if she doesn't, she deserves my anger.	That's placing too much power in the hands of one person, and too little responsibility in my own hands.
If I don't get angry, I'll be hurt again.	I can coolly and firmly stand up for my rights and may not need to be angry, or excessively angry.
If I can't control someone, I'll be out of control.	Since people have free agency, we can never really control someone else. We can only try to earn their respect and love.
Hitting her is the only way to get her off my back.	Other methods to try include respecting her, problem solving, listening, and humor.
If you hurt me, I am entitled to hurt you back.	This mindset keeps countries at war. I can become so strong inside that you don't have the power to hurt me, and I can sometimes try to reclaim you despite your behavior.

Core Beliefs	**Alternatives**
My self-esteem is at stake when my authority is challenged.	Your reputation with others might be at risk, but self-esteem is independent of others' opinions.
I must be in charge.	Shared control and trust is very useful and satisfying in relationships.
People must be punished.	People can be led.
People are bad.	People are a mixture of strengths and weaknesses.
I must be respected to be happy.	That would be nice, but I can choose happiness without it.
In order to be worthwhile, I must be better than others.	One's worth is not comparative.
I must be successful to be liked.	Many likeable people are not particularly success-ful or prestigious.
It's awful to be mediocre.	Half of all people are below average. Some of them are quite content.
I am weak.	I am a combination of weaknesses and strengths. I am strengthening the weaker areas.
My weaknesses/flaws will be exposed—how horrible!	Everyone is fallible; each person has flaws. To have them exposed makes me human. That's not awful, just life. Actually, some flaws are endearing.
If I am not respected by others, I have no value; I cease to exist.	Nobody's opinion determines my worth.
To lose control is awful.	Loss of control is inevitable. Many things in life are beyond my control. Sometimes all I can con-trol is the way I look at the loss of control. Paradoxically, to accept loss of control helps me control my stress. I *can* endure loss of control.
Bad things won't happen if I am good enough and careful enough.	Rain falls on the good, the bad, and the in-between. Some things happen randomly and are not indicative of divine disfavor. The best we can do is be prepared.

Table 4.8 (Continued)

Core Beliefs	Alternatives
I should judge and punish myself for my shortcomings and failings.	I can greet myself cordially and with encouragement—this is a better way to grow and develop. I'll leave the judgment to others.
My worth is diminished by mistakes.	My worth as a unique individual is far too complex to be reduced to isolated performances. Mistakes reflect our skill level or development at the time. A mistake does not totally and irrevocably define a person.
The best person always wins. So I must always win.	If that were true, championship teams would always be undefeated. I can try my best and then enjoy the outcome.

Now imagine that C, the emotional consequences, significantly changes so that you are now no longer seriously angry, but relatively calm; irritated, but not furious. Ask, "What thoughts changed in order to cause this shift in emotions?"

This imagery not only affords practice in staying calm, but also reinforces our ability to choose calming thoughts.

Role Reversal Exercise

Take an anger-promoting core belief that you often find yourself using. Have a partner argue for the reasonableness of that core belief, while you try to explain why that core belief is not very reasonable and not very beneficial.

Devil's Advocate

Have one person read one of the core beliefs from Table 4.8. Have several other people take turns providing various rational alternatives to that core belief. This is a very useful drill to reinforce your ability to quickly replace distorted core beliefs under pressure.

Drills

- When you encounter a hook, simply notice, without judging yourself, what you are telling yourself.
- Ask yourself if your self-talk is helping you to feel good.

Reflections

When a man cannot distinguish a great from a small event, he is of no use.

(Sir Winston Churchill)

The trivial errors of others don't require your preoccupation and correction.

(Meyer Friedman, M.D.)

Do not seek perfection in a changing world. Instead, perfect your love.

(*Buddha's Little Instruction Book*)

Suggested Activities

1. Each day for two weeks, select an upsetting event and complete a Daily Thought Record. You might start with a specific hook that you encountered recently and progress to past or future hooks.
2. For a week, use the question-and-answer technique once a day to determine your core beliefs. Use previously completed Daily Thought Records, or a newly completed Daily Thought Record.

3. Try rational emotive imagery, the role reversal exercise, or the devil's advocate exercise (described earlier) to reinforce your cool thinking skills.

4. Add these activities:

- From your Daily Thought Records, write down several reasonable responses on three-by-five-inch cards. Place these cards on your bathroom mirror, refrigerator, computer screen, or other frequented place of choice.
- In your journal, write about a negative core belief. You might consider where it came from and what it would be like if it were replaced by a more reasonable belief.

5

Self-Esteem

What others think of us would be of little moment did it not, when known, so deeply tinge what we think of ourselves.

—George Santayana

We need to see ourselves as basic miracles.

—Virginia Satir

STEVE WAS FUMING at the stinging criticism he received from his boss. Not only did it seem unfair, it also made him feel diminished as a person. A glance at the list of anger hooks in Exhibit 1.1 (page 9) reveals that many of the things that trigger anger threaten self-esteem—the sense of who we are. The more insecure and vulnerable we feel inside, the more likely we will be to perceive hooks as threatening and to react with anger. Conversely, the person with deep, stable self-esteem is less likely to be shaken or disturbed by the world's chaos and attacks.[1] So to learn how to manage and minimize anger, it makes sense to also understand self-esteem and how it may be strengthened.

About Self-Esteem

Self-esteem is defined simply as a realistic, appreciative opinion of oneself. *Realistic* means that we see ourselves accurately and honestly, neither inflating nor deflating our strengths or importance. *Appreciative* implies positive feelings of liking and accepting. The person with self-esteem is generally secure. *Secure* means free from fear and doubt; not troubled; stable; safe from damage or attack. Secure people are aware of their strengths and weaknesses, and are comfortable with who they are inside. They are deeply and quietly glad to be who they are. They are relatively safe from attack because they know deep inside that nothing anyone can do or say can change their abiding worth as a human being.

People with self-esteem have no need for arrogance or destructive pride—the belief that they are more worthwhile as a person than others, or more capable than they are. Arrogance and destructive pride lead to enmity and competition, rather than cooperation. They cause us to view people on a vertical scale—one must be above others in order to have worth. People with self-esteem also possess a dignified humility. They realize that at a very basic level they are like all people—wanting to be happy and avoid suffering. Like all others, they are born, they die, and they share the same bodily functions. They wish to be loved and respected, and feel the same feelings of gladness, sadness, fear, and anger. Thus, self-esteem views people on a level playing field, equally worthwhile as human beings and warranting respectful treatment.

The Pillars of Self-Esteem

Self-esteem is like a house resting on three pillars, or foundation stones: (1) unconditional worth, (2) unconditional love, and (3) growing. Self-esteem is built by laying these foundation stones securely in this important sequence. If one foundation stone is not in place, the structure falls.

Unconditional Worth

Unconditional worth is the recognition that all people have infinite, eternal, equal, unchanging worth as human beings. Unconditional worth is to be distinguished from market or social worth, which clearly can change and which varies from person to person. Unconditional worth goes much deeper. Consider a newborn baby. Like the seed of a flower, that baby possesses in embryo every attribute needed to flourish. Were that child to fall into a well, parents would spend untold effort and resources to rescue that child, not because of what the child had accomplished in the world, but because of the child's innate worth.

We also like to compare each person to a beautiful cut crystal. Each facet represents an attribute that all people have—the capacity to love, make fruitful decisions, create, have a sense of humor, elevate others, laugh, beautify, etc. These capacities exist in embryo.[2] Each person develops these skills in different ways and patterns, but each person has all the attributes needed to live well. For example, some people may manifest their creativity artistically, while other people may show it in the way they cope with stress, make people laugh, earn a living, or clean the house. In some people, creativity is relatively dormant for a long time, but then flourishes later in life. Mistakes, rejection, criticism, poverty, or disrespectful treatment—these are all externals that do not diminish the core worth of a person. Think of the crystal being covered by a dirty film. When so surrounded, the core self (represented by the crystal) does not shine, but the crystal's worth remains intact. Conversely, compliments, successes, love, respectful treatment, popularity, financial security—these are also externals. They are like a halo that shines and brightens the core. These do not increase core human worth, which is already infinite and unchanging. They only help us to experience our worth with more joy.

Again, the analogy of a newborn helps us to understand why each person has unconditional worth. A baby is pure potential. There is also something very lovable about each child—it is a thrill to see them laugh, discover nature's beauty, respond to love. Do they irritate us at times and make mistakes? Of course. Yet we love and treasure them just the same. That love gives them the security to grow. A similar attitude toward ourselves helps us to grow.

If one considers human worth to be unchanging, then self-esteem will not fluctuate with life's ups and downs. For example, if one equates one's worth as a person to one's portfolio or market worth, then self-esteem might rise and fall with the stock market. If one equates one's worth as a person to one's appearance, then self-esteem will fall as one ages or gains weight. It is satisfying and invigorating to maintain physical conditioning, but it is wise to separate core worth from one's appearance. Appearance and wealth are externals.

You might have noticed that many of the distortions of cognitive therapy (in Chapter 4) relate to threatened worth. For instance, a person might think, "It's awful to be wrong; I must be right," because being wrong is erroneously equated to diminished worth. Also, self-esteem is not image management. Core worth is independent of stylish clothes or the opinions of others (otherwise it would be *other*-esteem).

Unconditional Love

It is clear from the research that children who know they are loved develop stronger self-esteem. Parents who raise children with self-esteem are interested in their welfare. They spend time with them, talk to them, ask about their friends, accept their feelings, and provide discipline—kindly, calmly, and firmly. The sometimes unspoken message is: "I believe in you. I expect good things from you. I will listen to and respect your point of view. But I also know you are not perfect, so I will set reasonable limits to show that I care and to help you grow."

Love is like the watered soil that allows the seed to grow with secure roots. One cannot love too much. One can be too permissive or too controlling, but that is not love. The former gives the message "I don't care," while the latter says, "I don't trust you."

If one did not receive unconditional love from parents, then one can learn to provide such love to oneself. Love of self does not mean selfishness, which can be a protective response to insecurity and pain. Instead, wholesome love grows the inner strength and security that eventually enables people to look beyond themselves, to lose themselves in the service of others.

Unconditional love entails acceptance. To accept is to receive gladly. To accept children is to let them know that they are wanted and valued, and that they belong in their home. Feelings are honored and talked about, so that children learn to manage and be comfortable with all kinds of feelings.

Love is a natural feeling. Sometimes people become hardened by life experiences, but the capacity to love and be loved, though buried, is never extinguished. Love is also an attitude that wants what is best for the loved person at all times. Finally, love is a skill that is learned and cultivated—and a decision that we make every day (that is, we choose to love sometimes, even though we may not feel like it). Thus, we might think of loving as an innate capacity that can be cultivated.

Growing

Once people clearly see their unconditional human worth and love themselves despite their imperfections, they then possess the security needed to grow with joy. Growing is moving up the staircase toward full development of one's innate capacities. It is an ongoing process that is never fully completed. Yet if we know that we are moving in a desired direction, at the pace that is uniquely suited to each of us, then we can feel a deep satisfaction. Perfection is not required to have self-esteem. If so, no one would ever possess it. Do you know people who have achieved brilliantly but lack self-esteem? It is usually because they lack the foundation stones of unconditional worth and unconditional love. Without this security, they feel they must achieve in order to have worth. But achievement alone will never give one a feeling of at-homeness. Achievement does not establish core worth; it only reminds us of it and allows us to experience ourselves with greater satisfaction.

How does one grow? Simply by lifting oneself and others. The possibilities are infinite, which is why it is good to patiently enjoy the process and not become attached to the outcome. We can develop greater integrity/character (see Chapter 10). We can serve individuals or communities in countless ways. We can cultivate hobbies or talents that bring pleasure—not because they impress or provide a false sense of superiority. We can improve other abilities to experience wholesome pleasures (see Chapter 9). We can nurture our sense of humor or creativity.

Can Self-Esteem Change?

At the University of Maryland we have found that self-esteem can improve in a relatively short amount of time by learning and applying specific skills. In the interest of space, we will sample only some of these skills.

"Nevertheless"

People without self-esteem are easily threatened by stressful events because the events become a test of worth. They think, "Because I was criticized (was rejected, made a mistake, was treated rudely, etc.), therefore my worth is diminished."

Conversely, people with self-esteem know that core worth cannot be diminished, no matter what people do or say. So even though they might feel diminished, they quickly remind themselves that this is just a feeling, not reality. The "nevertheless" skill reinforces this belief. The format is:

> *Even though you criticized my performance* (you don't think much of me, you dumped me, I messed up, or some other statement of fact), *nevertheless I'm a worthwhile person.*

Notice, that this honestly acknowledges two realities: First, we are not perfect. Second, we are still worthwhile. Mistakes, criticism, rejection, etc., are externals that do not diminish core worth. If someone calls you a loser, you can use your cognitive therapy skills and think, "Even though you think that (or I didn't *perform* too well), nevertheless I'm a worthwhile person."

The "nevertheless" stem can also be completed with statements of love or growing. For example:

- Even though you treat me rudely, nevertheless I love myself.
- Even though I made a mistake, nevertheless I am growing (am trying to improve, have the right to try, etc.).

Acknowledging Strengths

To be quietly aware of and appreciative of your unique strengths is not boasting. Rather it is a skill that builds inner security and quiet confidence. Are you or have you ever been *reasonably* clean, handy, dependable, adventurous, organized, industrious, flexible, friendly, resourceful, or persistent? Are you sometimes a *reasonably* good socializer, listener, cook, follower, leader, supporter, worker, driver, or helper? Although no one is perfect, each person has a unique combination or pattern of strengths. It is good to remind ourselves from time to time of what is presently right about ourselves. The following skill is based on the research of three Canadian psychologists, Gauthier, Pellerin, and Renaud, whose method improved the self-esteem of subjects in just a few weeks.[3]

Cognitive Rehearsal

- Develop a list of ten strengths you possess—attributes that are meaningful and true. Rather than identifying roles (such as "I am a good real estate agent"), try to identify personal characteristics ("I understand people"). Roles can change (one could retire or be fired), but characteristics are enduring.

- Find a quiet, relaxing place. Look at one statement, then meditate on the evidence for the accuracy of that statement for a minute or two. Repeat this for each of the ten statements. For example, "As a real estate agent, I can tune in to people's unspoken needs. I am good at helping them meet those needs in a respectful way." This will take about fifteen to twenty minutes altogether.

- Repeat this for ten days. Instead of meditating on all the statements during one session, you might prefer to place the statements on separate index cards and carry the cards with you. Throughout the day, pull out one card at a time. Look at the strength and reflect upon the evidence for its accuracy for a minute or two.

Acknowledging Hurt and Insecurity

It is painful to feel insecure and vulnerable. Yet everyone feels this way at times. Sometimes to protect ourselves from these painful feelings, we become angry. One woman confessed, "I like to make people afraid of me—it protects me." In other words, she was using anger to defend against feeling pain. Of course, anger just keeps things the way they are. No healing takes place. Paradoxically, one of the best ways to heal insecurity is to acknowledge that it exists. Feelings make us human. To shut down some of those feelings is to reject who we are. To accept the full range of emotions is to accept ourselves fully. The next time you notice anger beginning to swell, try thinking, "Okay, I'm getting angry, and what I'm also feeling is . . . . That's okay. That's life." Feeling insecure (or afraid, vulnerable, hurt, lonely, sad, or anything else) makes you human and fallible, not less worthwhile. Accepting yourself despite having uncomfortable feelings does not equate to complacency or unwillingness to resolve those feelings. Recall the principle: Love provides the foundation of growth. Condemning oneself is of no benefit whatsoever. Once we acknowledge insecurities and pain in ourselves, we will find it easier to be compassionate to others who are struggling or offensive.

If you are willing to risk it, try confiding your real feelings (i.e., those that are beneath the anger) occasionally to people you trust. They might feel relief to know that you feel such feelings, too. They might even like you better knowing that you are vulnerable. Emotionally mature people will not use this against you. If they do, practice your "nevertheless" skill.

Fallibility Antidotes

Dr. Seuss wrote a wonderful book called *Oh, the Places You'll Go*. It essentially says that you will go far, except when you don't, because sometimes you won't. And people will really like you, except when they don't, because sometimes they won't. There is an art to failing without allowing it to erode self-esteem. The following are some helpful principles:

- *Talk or write about it.* Putting words down on paper helps to release the feeling of failure, provides perspective, and permits time to make sense of what happened.

- *Accurately assign responsibility.* Accept appropriate responsibility. Acknowledge where you were wrong or mistaken. Also acknowledge extenuating circumstances or contributing factors. ("This was a very difficult situation. I was inexperienced, tired, under pressure to make a quick decision.")

- *Rate behavior, not the core.* People are too complex for simplistic labels such as "loser." They are more than their mistakes. Reject behaviors, but accept people.

- *Replace the word* failure *with words such as* setback, mistake, falling short, *or* learning experience.

- *View the fallible self with compassion and acceptance.* Fallible does not mean worthless.

- *Accept the outcome, but maintain an optimistic focus.* View the mistake as a building block, not a stumbling block. You might think, "Okay, it happened. Now, what have I learned? What behaviors will I change in the future?"

- *Realize that ascent is difficult.* It takes repeated efforts. Since fallibility is an inescapable aspect of life, expect slips from time to time.

- *Take your knocks and move on.* Most people will forget about it. You might as well, too.

Drill

Look in the mirror. Instead of noticing imperfections, look into your eyes with genuine understanding and compassion.

Reflections

I am no more important than the person who is offending me. Neither am I less important.

(Anonymous)

Each of us must work for his own improvement, and at the same time share general responsibility for all humanity.

(Marie Curie)

No one really knows enough to be a pessimist.

(Norman Cousins)

A human being's first responsibility is to shake hands with himself.

(Henry Winkler)

Suggested Activities

1. Several times a day, try the "nevertheless" skill for upsetting events in this order: First try a "nevertheless I'm a worthwhile person" response until that becomes automatic. Then try a "nevertheless I love me" statement until automatic. Then try growing statements.
2. Practice the cognitive rehearsal skill (page 105) over a ten-day period.
3. In your journal, continue to explore the feelings beneath your anger in an accepting, compassionate way.

6

Meditation

*Every breath we take, every step we make, can be filled
with peace, joy, and serenity. We need only to be awake,
alive in the present moment.*

—Thich Nhat Hanh

MEDITATION IS A very well-researched form of relaxation. It first
calms the mind, and then the body follows. Harvard's Dr. Herbert
Benson has noted that four to six weeks of practice typically results
in reductions in stress, short temper, headaches, backaches, insomnia, cholesterol levels, blood pressure, hyperventilation, anxiety, and
panic attacks; and in enhanced creativity.[1] *More than a relaxation
strategy, however, meditation also cultivates a new attitude toward
the self, others, and life, which can result in greater inner peace,
security, and empathy.*

Because meditation has been recorded in Eastern and Western
cultures throughout history, it is described somewhat differently by
different people. I'd like to present it as I have come to understand it,
recognizing that there are many other ways to teach it. For years I
taught meditation in the rather scientific way that Dr. Benson teaches
it. I still do. However, I have also incorporated the perspectives of
Tibetan masters, for several reasons. First, it makes the experience

richer by providing a simple way to look at human nature and growth. Second, the Tibetan approach is respectful of, and easily harmonized with, other philosophical approaches, including Judeo–Christian perspectives and Western psychology. Third, although I am not a Buddhist, I have come to respect the character and teachings of the Tibetan leaders, and find them quite consistent with my teachings. For example, after China overran Tibet, killing more than a million people and destroying thousands of beautiful temples and monasteries, the spiritual leaders have peacefully and without hatred worked to reclaim their homeland. They harbor no bitterness for the Chinese, while condemning their behavior. When we practice meditation we can incorporate such perspectives if it seems helpful, or none at all if that is desired.

What Is Meditation?

Meditation is awareness of one's true, happy nature. My first teacher taught that one need not fight fear; one need only be aware of love. One need not flee pain; one need only penetrate it with peaceful awareness, without fear or avoidance. When we create a safe environment we often discover inner strengths that have previously been untapped in the flurry of busy modern living. Sometimes we become aware of hurts that need to be healed with kindness. Sometimes we discover insights. For example, the Buddhists describe a gopher that is being chased by a lion that is interested in a meal. The gopher jumps off a cliff. While falling, the gopher notices a bear below, its mouth wide open, so it grabs a root on the side of the cliff. Dangling there, between the lion and the bear, the gopher notices a flower. It reaches over, takes a bite, and says, "How delicious!" The lesson, of course, is that even amidst moments of chaos there exist potential moments of joy, if one has eyes to see. We can find joy in pleasure or pain, as life offers.

What Is Meditating Like?

Recall a time that was very pleasant. Perhaps you think of a sunset on the ocean. Perhaps you think of holding a sleeping child or a loved one. What such moments have in common is that you were pleasantly absorbed in the moment, peacefully aware. Your attention was not pulled away or distracted by worries.

Tibetan masters teach that when water in a glass is agitated, it is not clear. As the water settles, it becomes clear. Meditation allows the mind to settle, see clearly, and pleasantly dance or play with whatever arises.

Meditation only requires a quiet place to practice, a comfortably alert posture, a point on which to focus concentration (be it the breath, a calming word, or a prayer), and a passive attitude that pleasantly accepts whatever happens. Although there are many ways to meditate, the techniques are not the same as the experience. That is, the various methods can all help us to feel a peaceful, settled clarity and a greater sense of security.

Wisdom Mind, Ordinary Mind

Sogyal Rinpoche teaches that we have two minds—the wisdom mind (sometimes called the essential, serene mind) and the ordinary mind (sometimes called the nonessential, superficial mind).[2] (See Figure 6.1.)

Figure 6.1 Two Minds

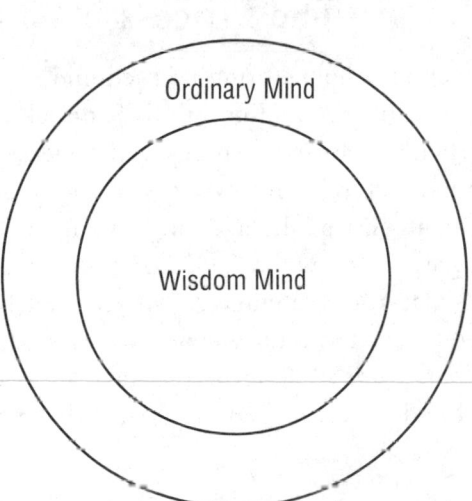

The wisdom mind represents your true, happy nature—uncomplicated and clear. The wisdom mind is wise and benevolent. It is happy because it desires the happiness of others as much as your own. It has calm, peaceful emotions. It is joyful, good humored, loving, and accepting. It has dignity, self-esteem, and humility. It is also flexible, hopeful, and expansive in scope. It is where the various fragments of the self dissolve and unify as friends.

The ordinary mind surrounds and walls off the wisdom mind. It keeps you ignorant of your happy nature and causes many problems and suffering. The ordinary mind grasps and attaches to things that are illusory or unimportant, such as greed, false fronts, and pride, which leads to hurt and jealousy. The ordinary mind is marked by disturbing negative emotions, such as sorrow, worry, anger in all its forms, ignorance, and confusion. It is not integrated, but is scattered and restless. When people say they are beside themselves with anger, they mean that they are pulled away from their wisdom mind.

Rinpoche explains that enlightenment occurs when we realize or glimpse our true nature. The light of this true nature bursts forth, shatters the walls of the ordinary mind, and merges with the greater light and truth beyond. In moving beyond your own unwanted tendencies to hurt and be negative (the ordinary mind), you then are able to connect with and serve others. And this is a root of happiness.

The Process

Meditation is feeling at home, bringing the mind, which is scattered and beaten, to rest in the wisdom mind. Rinpoche teaches one to "release and relax."[3] Release graspings and nonessential aspects of the ordinary mind, and relax into your true, happy nature. Imagine that you have spent a crisp fall day laboring outside. Perhaps you've been raking leaves, piling wood, and doing every needful thing to beautify your yard. You've completed all you had hoped to do, so you're completely relaxed and without worries as you go inside. After a warm bath, you settle into your favorite overstuffed chair, deeply satisfied and peaceful. You are aware that you, like all others, possess a wisdom mind, just as all people possess a core of unconditional worth.

Physical Preparation

Rinpoche likens the posture in meditation to a mountain. A mountain is dignified, profoundly stable, and secure. It is always the same, despite the winds, rain, snow, clouds, or darkness that buffet or surround it. At the peak, the mountain commands an expansive view that compassionately sees into the hearts of all people who are suffering and want to be happy.[4] The back is straight—you might imagine the spine filled with light. The chest and shoulders hold a poised, yet tensionless posture. I think of Sarah Brightman in concert. Originally trained as a dancer, she at times holds her hands together in front of her body with a dignified grace that is poised, yet relaxed.

The eyes are closed so that visual stimuli do not interfere with the peaceful experience. The hands rest in the lap. Some like to comfortably cover their knees with their hands. Others prefer to rest them palms down in the lap. I prefer to rest them palms up in the lap; any choice is appropriate. The attitude is one of gentle amusement, brightness, humility, and self-esteem, which arises from the awareness that we all have a true happy nature.

How to Rest the Mind

A small portion of your attention is focused gently on the breath and a calming word as a way of relaxing into the wisdom mind. Notice the calming aspects of the breath. The calming word is a *mantra*, or word that peacefully distracts from the negativity of the ordinary mind and settles you into the restful wholeness of the wisdom mind. While focusing on the breath and the mantra, you just allow your mind to rest blissfully. As quiet water becomes clear, so too your mind becomes clear. Swirling thoughts begin to settle.

There are a number of ways to handle worries that arise and can pull you out of the wisdom mind. All of these ways have great utility for handling fears in everyday life. Rinpoche suggests that you watch them as an old man watches a child at play, or as we would watch clouds moving across the sky. He also likens an intrusive thought to a small wave that arises in the midst of a vast ocean, and then recedes back into that great body of water. Finally, you might imagine yourself standing by the railing of a riverboat, enjoying the beautiful view. Soon a log floats down the river into your view. You could think, "I don't like that old log spoiling my view. I shall jump into the water and wrestle with it." This, of course, would ruin your experience and not very effectively remove the log from view. Instead, you could simply notice the log float into view, let it float on by, think, "That's okay, that's life," and then return your awareness to the beautiful scenery. Similarly, we can greet worries cordially, let them pass through awareness, and let the mantra ride in behind them into awareness.

In meditation, the mind is both alert and relaxed, without attempting to be too solemn. Because a few minutes of mindful clarity is more valuable than longer periods of distracted focus, beginners start with just a few minutes of meditation, progressing over time to ten- to twenty-minute sessions. If your practice is not effective and your mind wanders, take a break. Just sit quietly for a few moments before returning to the practice of meditating. All attempts are useful, so just be gentle and pleasantly accept whatever happens.

When you meditate, it helps to remind yourself that it is okay not to be achieving for a few moments. In fact, resting helps people to live and produce more effectively. Patiently look for quiet moments of peace, not drama or fireworks. Just as a simple meal can be very satisfying if it is peaceful and pleasant, so can a simple period of meditation be satisfying and peaceful.

Meditation Instructions

1. Get comfortable. Remove glasses or contact lens. Loosen tight clothing and remove shoes, if desired.

2. To prepare for meditation, stand up. Spread your feet to approximately shoulder width. As you breathe in, imagine the sun

evaporating the earth's moisture and forming clouds as you raise your hands up toward the ceiling. Exhaling, let your fingers dance and fall to your sides as you imagine rain blanketing the earth. Inhaling, grasp your hands together behind you. Exhaling, bend over, forming a rainbow that smiles over the earth (don't forget to smile). Inhaling, straighten up. Exhaling, let your arms fall to your sides. Inhaling, raise your hands and arms up to shoulder level in front of you, as you greet the rising sun. Exhaling, embrace the sun by bringing your hands together, forming a circle with your arms and hands. Feel the warmth. Inhaling, draw the warmth of the sun inside you by bringing your hands to your heart. Exhaling, feel the warmth inside you.[5]

3. Sit comfortably in a chair, with your feet flat on the floor and your hands resting in your lap. Use the whole back of the chair to support your spine, sitting comfortably erect. You might first slump forward in your chair. Then imagine a hook on the crown of your head. A string pulls that hook straight up toward the ceiling. As this is done, the spine straightens but without needless tension in the body. The shoulders, neck, and jaw are relaxed. Think of the dignified mountain, which is unshakable, majestic, at ease with itself despite the winds and rains that batter it.

4. Allow your eyes to close with an attitude of optimism, playfulness, humility, and self-esteem.

5. Release and relax into your mind. Imagine returning from a hard day's labor in the garden. You've done all you set out to do; there is nothing left to do or worry about. So you release your cares, settle into a soft chair, and relax into your mind.

6. Relax your whole body. Release tension starting with your feet, legs, stomach, chest, back, shoulders, arms, and hands. Relax your neck, scalp, forehead, eyes, jaw, and mouth.

7. Take two easy, deep breaths, saying your calming word or phrase to yourself as you breathe in and as you breathe out.

8. Breathe abdominally, normally, paying attention to the calming rhythm of the breath. On the in-breath notice the gentle coolness of the air. On the out-breath notice the pleasant, relaxing feeling as air is expelled and the chest sinks down gently. As you concentrate on your breathing, perhaps you notice that external stimulation fades, much like the roar of the waves seems to fade after you have been on the beach for a while. You might notice that breathing slows of its own accord and becomes more rhythmic as you peacefully watch whatever happens.

9. Thinking of waves gently ebbing and flowing from the shore, let your mind ride the waves of the in-breath. (Pause) Let your mind ride the waves of the out-breath. (Pause) As your mind settles in the breath, it slows and becomes clear.

10. Begin to concentrate on the word "One" rolling in on the in-breath. Say silently and slowly on the in-breath, "One." After a few moments, begin to think of the word "One" rolling out on the out-breath.

11. Should distracting thoughts arise, greet them cordially. "That's okay, that's life." Let them float through your mind like clouds floating across the sky, as your mantra, "One," floats in and out on the in-breath and out-breath. Let the word "One" gently reverberate and roll around in your mind, filling your mind, allowing your breath, mantra, and awareness to become one, as you release and relax into your true happy nature for the next few moments.

Drill

Since meditation is an experience, more than a method, use various stimuli to remind you to release and relax into your true happy nature: a beautiful scene in nature, a smile, a greeting, a joke, a good book, driving, a picture, walking, or a phone call from a friend.

Reflections

Seeing into darkness is clarity.

(Lao Tzu, Chinese, c 600 B.C.)

Anger, violence, and aggression . . . arise when we are
frustrated in our efforts to achieve love and affection.
They are not part of our most basic, underlying nature.

(Dalai Lama)

Come back to the present moment and find peace and joy.

(Thich Nhat Hanh)

Words may help you understand something. Experience
allows you to know.

(Neale Donald Walsh)

Peace must first be developed within an individual.

(Dalai Lama)

Suggested Activity

You'll probably wish to practice meditating several times over the
course of the next few weeks, since the effectiveness of meditation
increases with repetition.

7

Variations on Meditation

I am the infinite deep . . . forever still.

—Ashtavakra Gita, Hindu Master

For God hath not given us the spirit of fear, but of power, and of love, and of a sound mind.

—2 Tim. 1:7

RECALL THAT MEDITATION can be a very effective way to calm the mind and the body, and that it can also grow many of the attitudes that are so important to anger management. This chapter will explore meditation variations that further promote inner strength, security, and calmness so that you'll be less reactive to potential provocations.

These variations are generally short, so they can be practiced frequently during the day without major adjustments in lifestyle. For example, you might try them upon awakening, during work breaks, or on the bus or train.

Inner Strength and Self-Soothing Meditation

This very soothing, brief meditation was developed by McNeal and Frederick:[1]

> As you pay attention to your breathing, you can notice that in between each inhalation there is a moment of quiet space . . . and you know that you have within you this same quiet space . . . It's a place that feels like the very center of your being, that place where it's very quiet and peaceful and still . . . And in this place you can just take a few moments and enjoy the sensation of breathing in and breathing out . . . how good it feels . . . and you can enjoy how good your whole body feels . . . your arms . . . your legs . . . your trunk . . . how wonderful it is now just to take a breath and let it out . . . and just the way you can enjoy that comfort in your body . . . you can let yourself feel now . . . a deep peacefulness of your spirit . . . your feelings . . . It's even possible that you may notice that certain images will float into your mind that are beautiful or especially comforting to you . . . in this peaceful . . . calm . . . special place inside you.
>
> [This ability to find inner peace is a great inner strength.] When you're in touch with this part of yourself, it's possible to feel more calm—knowing you have the capacity to calm and soothe yourself and parts of yourself that have needed this calming and soothing so much.

You might enhance the effectiveness of this meditation by ending with two deep, cleansing breaths. At first, take a deep, quiet abdominal breath, filling an imaginary balloon under the navel with air. When the balloon is full, let the wave of the in-breath gradually fill your lower lungs, and then the middle and upper lungs. Keep your shoulders relaxed and still throughout. As you prepare to exhale, notice your heartbeat. As you exhale, let the out-breath carry all tension and strain from your heart as your heartbeat becomes calm, quiet, and steady. Take another deep cleansing breath. First fill the balloon, then let the wave of inhalation gradually fill the lungs. As you prepare to exhale, think of your mind and brain. As you exhale, let your mind become very calm and clear as you release all needless concerns.

Constructive Power Meditation

We all feel powerless and out of control at times. No one likes to feel that way. As we do, anger can arise as an expression of pain and an attempt to regain power. The more powerless one feels, the more likely anger is to become excessive and destructive. Think of a child in a poor neighborhood who joins a violent gang to overcome feelings of fear, weakness, and isolation. Now think of a man who cannot seem to win the love and respect of his wife, so he turns to violence in order to control her. Or an office worker who destroys her computer in frustration. In these examples, destructive power attempts to compensate for the apparent lack of constructive power. However, destructive power does not feel peaceful, is costly, and does not address our deepest needs. It is a counterfeit type of power that hides the real hurt and thus prevents us from healing. At best, it only temporarily numbs the pain of feeling powerless. It provides no genuine control and is not true to our best self. Although we do not have the power to change other people and certain situations, even prisoners of war have great power in some respects. That is, when their external freedoms are taken away, they discover the capacity to develop their inner lives.

An antidote to a sense of powerlessness is connecting to the *internal constructive* power of our true core selves. Experiencing this strong inner power enables us to see ourselves as strong and calm. This will enable us to stay calmer during those times when outer circumstances can't be controlled.

Here we shall meditate on our true, constructively powerful nature, realizing that we are generally capable of much strength and control. This helps us accept the inevitable loss of control in certain situations without losing our sense of peace and constructive power.

Reflect on the ways in which you have *constructive* power. Place a check beside the items below that apply to you. *I have the strength inside to . . .*

- ☐ Know that my worth is not changed, even by the silly behavior or opinions of others
- ☐ Stay calm inside despite loss of control over outer events

- ☐ Not react at all to provocations

- ☐ Do the turtle trick—going within to reconnect to calmness and peace (see page 214)

- ☐ Locate resources; seek someone who has the needed skills that I lack at the moment

- ☐ Change the way I think about something that's disagreeable

- ☐ Calmly but firmly reason with others

- ☐ Exercise willpower—the power to firmly and calmly persist

- ☐ Take a break

- ☐ Love

- ☐ Learn, grow, laugh, play, and work

- ☐ Show compassion for people, though not necessarily their behavior

- ☐ Contribute to the elevation of others

- ☐ Treat all people with respect and kindness, even those I don't like

- ☐ Serve for the sake of others (and not worry about my own status)

- ☐ Create and beautify

- ☐ Return kindness for offenses ("I won't hurt or control you even if you choose to do that to me.")

- ☐ Release bitterness so that neither I nor the offender suffer more

- ☐ Make choices that are in my best interest and the best interest of others

- ☐ Discern the character of others

☐ Accept people despite their imperfections

☐ Acknowledge and accept my strengths and weaknesses

☐ Confront my own limitations

☐ Let go of the person I've been in order to become a better person

☐ Have character

☐ Retain my power within (i.e., not let others dictate my peace)

☐ Set, progress toward, and achieve reasonable goals

☐ Gain knowledge and understanding

☐ Overcome adversity

☐ Be true to my best self/principles, despite the treatment of others

☐ Be flexible when I don't get my way ("Okay, what's another way?")

☐ Learn new skills

☐ Heal the hurts that underlie my anger; rather than displacing my pain on others, I show myself extra respect and compassion when others offend me

☐ Optimize enjoyment in imperfect circumstances

☐ Improve my appearance

☐ Love the offender while sticking up for my right to respectful treatment; return firmness for offense

☐ Pray and place ultimate trust in God

☐ Discipline a child without anger or malice

Meditate on being so strong and powerful, in control, worthwhile, and happy that the times of loss of control and powerlessness become acceptable.

Core Worth Meditation

1. Think of a time when you felt connected to your core worth. This might include times when you:

- Were in the presence of someone who made you feel loved, respected, like a somebody
- Accomplished something of which you were wholesomely proud
- Were photographed, and the picture captured your inner brightness, joy, character, etc.
- Lovingly held a baby or watched one sleep
- Were dressed nicely and felt good
- Were treated with kindness and compassion
- Were uplifted by art, a movie, television, music, a cathedral, etc.
- Felt close to God (e.g., a child innocently praying)
- Did something brave or courageous
- Admitted a wrong and took responsibility to correct it
- Stood up for somebody who was weak or defenseless

2. Meditate on one of the instances you identified. Make the meditation as vivid as possible by recalling as many details of the event as you can—sights, sounds, smells, tactile sensations, emotions, inner states of the body.

3. This meditation can be repeated frequently, either with the same event or with others. Repeated practice reinforces the feelings of unconditional worth and unconditional love.

Confronting Wounds to Discover Strength Meditation

Anger temporarily numbs the pain but prevents healing. It is much like using alcohol to cover the pain, but the drunken state prevents healing. This meditation goes to the source of the anger so that the pain may be healed.

Think of something that angers you. Think of the pain that underlies the anger. Locate that pain in your body. Give it a color and shape. Go into the pain. Stay with it. Keep persisting, penetrating the pain, until you discover your strength. Stay with the darkness until you discover your light, clarity, peace, and strength.

I once listened to an oncologist, Dr. Rachel Naomi Remen, describe her interaction with a woman with cancer. The woman was frantically running around filling every minute of her day with activity, as a means to escape her fear of death. Dr. Remen asked the woman to calmly imagine the cancer in her body. The woman envisioned a dark shape in her body. Dr. Remen persisted in asking the woman to penetrate that darkness. At first the experience was frightening, but the woman persisted. Eventually, the darkness gave way to light, and the woman discovered inside herself an inner reserve of peace and strength that was larger than her fear. Thereafter her compulsive activity gave way to a calm security.

Reducing Reactivity to Angry People: The Feelings Dial Meditation

Some people react intensely to facial expressions in other people that convey disapproval, contempt, rejection, scorn, anger, etc. This overreaction may reflect a nervous system that is sensitized by previous experiences. This exercise will help to desensitize a nervous system that habitually overreacts to other people.

Think back to a time when someone treated you in such a way that you felt very angry or hurt. Perhaps you were criticized or treated with contempt. See the person's face and let yourself feel some of those upsetting feelings—the hurt, the pain, the anger.

Now imagine a "feelings" dial—like a volume dial on a radio—that represents how disturbed you feel as you look at the person's face. Imagine that 10 means the volume is turned all the way up, to extremely intense discomfort; 0 means there is no disturbance at all.

What number reflects how weak or strong your feelings are on the feelings dial? What would it be at 8? At 1? How about somewhere in the middle? If you'd like to try turning down the feelings dial, what number would you turn it to? Turn down the dial lower and lower until it goes down a number. And keep turning it lower and lower and lower. Would you like to keep going? Keep going nice and slow until you reach the desired level. You might use your easy deep breaths, and as you exhale, turn down the dial further. As you turn the dial down, your feelings and thoughts become calmer. You realize that you are actually regulating your level of reactivity. Notice that you can also turn the feelings dial up to any level you choose. For example, if you were feeling grief and anger, and had reduced the level to 1 on the feelings dial, you might decide that 3 is a good level. Here you can empathize and appropriately respond to others, but not be overwhelmed or controlled by your feelings. You really can turn your reaction to this person up or down, to whatever level you choose.

You also realize that no matter whom you come in contact with, no matter how disagreeable or contemptuous, you can look at the person's face, turn down the dial, and react at the level you choose.

Soothing, Wise Warrior Meditation

Anger can have an on–off quality, as if there is a part of us that erupts. This is a meditation to merge the angry, vulnerable self with the calm, logical self in a wholesome way, so that you'll behave in a more integrated, consistent manner.

Perhaps there is a part of you that is like a strong, protective warrior: angry, perhaps often or most of the time. See that part of you in imagery, having fought and survived many battles. Imagine now that the war has ended for a season—and that feels good.

Imagine that the warrior is now being welcomed home after years of battle, welcomed into the larger community with great appreciation and affection. You're glad to welcome that strong part of you. Send respect and love and gratitude for the way your warrior side has steadfastly tried to protect your interests. You might imagine sending a warm thank-you note or similar expression of gratitude. Observe that the warrior has grown somewhat older, stronger, wiser, more compassionate, and seems ready for a new job, an expanded role—to live peacefully in the community and protect all who are there in new ways. Laying down the weapons of war, knowing that they can be accessed again if needed, the warrior now selects the new tools of living: calmness . . . inner security . . . respect . . . resolute firmness . . . kindness . . . and protective, soothing love. The warrior seems content and eager to use these tools.

Drills

- Practice periods of silence (e.g., turn off the TV or radio). Begin with five to ten minutes, then work up to longer periods of time.
- When sitting in traffic or when you are kept waiting, allow the mind to wander. Ponder something pleasant: the scenery around you, faces, pleasant memories, what you are grateful for, an anticipated vacation, etc.

Reflections

A mind without anger is cool, fresh, and sane.

(Thich Nhat Hanh)

The soul craves depth of reflection.

(Thomas Moore)

Suggested Activity

Try the above meditations in place of or in combination with the basic wisdom mind meditation. For example, you might try one of the above meditations after doing the basic meditation for about ten minutes.

8

Hot Buttons:
Healing Hidden Wounds
from the Past

That which is not worked out will be acted out.

—John Bradshaw[1]

TELEVISION'S MR. (FRED) ROGERS received the 2001 Mental Health Award for helping to improve the nation's mental health.[2] He has observed, profoundly, that "Anything that's human is mentionable, and anything that's mentionable can be more manageable. Don't you often find that just having a good listener makes your upsetting times more manageable? When we can talk about our feelings, they can become less overwhelming, less upsetting, and less scary. The people we trust with that important talk can help us know that we're not alone and that our feelings are natural and normal."[3] The fortunate child grows up in a climate of emotional safety and respect, where all feelings can be acknowledged, discussed, and resolved. The child learns that sometimes we get angry even with those we love, and there are ways to express those feelings that don't hurt others. Developing an emotional vocabulary aids in the appropriate expression of feelings. Thus, Rogers continues, family members might appropriately acknowledge, "We were really angry with each other, weren't we?"[4] This does not mean that the love between family members is diminished. The wise parent communicates to the child, "It is permissible to cry; to feel sad, afraid, or angry—I'm here for you." Children from such families likely mature to the point that they live in the present without unresolved emotional baggage, having acquired a comfort with emotions, the skills to appropriately defuse them, and an intact sense of self.

But what happens when one carries wounds from the past that have not been expressed and resolved, and so never healed?

• Annie's father was an austere disciplinarian. As a child, she watched a friend run to her father's arms and embrace him. When she tried that with her father, he shook his finger and scolded, "You little stinker. What are you up to?" Decades later, she reflected with a curious mixture of anger and sadness, "I never tried to show him affection after that. He was such a stern man."

• Without discussion, Hal's parents insisted that he join the family business, although Hal had a strong desire to pursue his talent for music. Years later, he felt resentment toward his parents, and regret and disappointment toward himself.

• Maria's third child died at birth. She said, "I'm angry. I find it difficult to believe in a God who would let that happen." In her hurt, she shut down her spiritual feelings, which had previously provided her with much comfort.[5]

• Barry was only six when his father died. To protect him, his mother sent him to relatives during the funeral. He was never permitted to grieve his loss. He was taught never to express anger and to cover sadness with a smile. As an adult, he suffered from depression and hypertension. In later years, he became increasingly angry, reacting more and more to rather minor irritations. Rather than address the hurt, Barry's younger brother would try to deflect it with humor ("My, you're becoming forceful.").

• Anger expert Bradley Barris relates that his salty grandmother had divorced her nasty husband Charley. Fifty years later when something really irritated her (Charley was long deceased at this point), Grambo—as he called her—would shout, "Charley, you SOB!"[6]

• Wanda and Jean were raised in a reasonably functional family. The parents were struggling in a family business and were frequently away at work. Wanda, the oldest, was the "good girl," the responsible one. Jean, a middle child, felt unwanted and unappreciated. She viewed Wanda more as a caretaker, and not the respectful confidant she desired. Wanda couldn't understand Jean's sometimes immature attempts to gain attention and respect. As adults, they were cordial, but lacked a day-to-day warm relationship. Jean committed to come to her nephew's birthday party, but found a last-minute excuse. Wanda was angry that Jean would again be so irresponsible. Said Wanda, "I'd like to address my feelings, but I know I can't. When I've tried, Jean brings up hurts from thirty years ago and arguments make the relationship worse. I guess the relationship will never really get better. I try to ignore the problem, put it out of my head. Sometimes it helps, but then things like the party happen and I seethe with anger."

• Javier goes ballistic when he gets lost. He logically knows it is ridiculous to do so. He doesn't connect his reaction to times when he was left alone as a child and felt helpless and afraid.

• Wounds can also be caused by abuse (sexual, physical, or emotional), neglect, or other disturbing life experiences. For instance, a child might be sexually abused by a father, and then told to keep it a secret, lest she cause the breakup of the family. Or a neighbor threatens to kill a child if she reveals sexual abuse. In either case, the confusing feelings are locked in memory—unexpressed and unresolved.

For various reasons, the individuals in the examples above were not able to express and/or work through their hurts in an accepting emotional environment. It becomes evident that unhealed emotional wounds can affect the present in many ways.

1. *Anger*. Buried, unresolved anger smolders and can easily be ignited. It is as though hot buttons in the present are wired to wounds from the past. We might encounter hooks that are vaguely reminiscent of past hurts. Though different on the surface, the hook might trigger feelings that are similar to the deeper wounds of the

past. We'd wish to think that such issues are long forgotten. We might not even be aware of festering anger or hurt. Nevertheless, we erupt "inexplicably" at rather "silly" hooks. However, a good look reveals that the eruption really isn't inexplicable and the hurt isn't so silly at all.

2. *Other troubling emotions*. Because anger rarely occurs alone, unhealed wounds can also lead to depression, worry, anxiety, panic attacks, and/or post-traumatic stress disorder.

3. *Medical illness*. Shakespeare wisely observed that unspoken emotional wounds might be expressed as physical illness. Recent research indicates that inhibited emotional expression is associated with disorders of the respiratory, digestive, cardiovascular, and endocrine systems.

Is there a way to defuse past situations that fuel present anger? Are there ways to go back, lovingly touch the hurt, and heal the fearful child that is beneath the anger? How do we heal the wound, when the offense or the offender doesn't change? Are there deeper salves, when here-and-now skills are not sufficient? How do we process old wounds so that we can move beyond them?

Confiding Hidden Wounds

Dr. James W. Pennebaker, a psychologist at University of Texas at Austin, has conducted an intriguing line of research to address such questions.[7] He has found that so-called "normal" adults carry a surprising range of unresolved wounds around with them. Childhood wounds are least likely to be confided, and adults are especially vulnerable to illness when such wounds have not been confided. Conversely, when adults were given the opportunity to confide their secret wounds in writing, for fifteen to thirty minutes a day for four days, some remarkable changes occurred. The mood initially slipped during the four days of writing. Some cried as they wrote or had dreams about the past events. They often reported that they understood their experience better after writing; it no longer hurt as much to think about it. After the four days of writing, confiders felt happier and less anxious than subjects in a control group who simply wrote about insignificant aspects of their childhoods. The confiders were also healthier, got sick less often, and had stronger immune systems.

Pennebaker investigated Holocaust survivors, survivors of the death of a spouse, and people who got fired from their jobs, concluding that confiding is healthy. It seems to help people confront, understand, and organize traumas. For example, fired employees who confided in writing were two to five times more likely to find new jobs, perhaps because they were less angry in their job interviews. Confiding seems to help hostile people.

Research has found that talking to a therapist or into a tape recorder provides similar benefits to writing. The key component of confiding seems to be that people verbalize the facts *and* feelings of difficult experiences. Verbalizing (especially in writing, which slows down the thought process) seems to integrate fragments of difficult memories and facilitate understanding (much like teaching helps the teacher to understand complex subject material). Verbalizing also literally expresses (i.e., discharges) distressing feelings. The process is done in a nonjudgmental way that accepts feelings, so that we can make sense of them.

Avoiding feelings keeps those feelings unprocessed and unhealed. It takes great energy to suppress distressing emotions, which perhaps explains why disclosers have fewer illnesses. People might try to avoid distressing feelings by working or exercising compulsively, denying that they are hurting, avoiding talking about the hurt, intellectualizing (sometimes worrying is just a way to think about a fear without feeling), or becoming angry (which covers the underlying feelings).

It is not surprising that people would instinctively try to avoid distressing feelings. First, those feelings, by definition, are uncomfortable. It is natural to wish to avoid suffering. People might fear that distressing feelings will overwhelm them and prevent them from coping in the present. They might not have learned to express feelings appropriately, or worse, been taught that it was weak or futile to feel distressing feelings. However, avoidance keeps things as they are.

Writing about all the feelings surrounding an event overcomes avoidance. Remember that accepting the full range of feelings is a way to wholesomely accept who you are and to heal. Once we set the healing process in motion, the mind has a greater chance to heal itself. Rather than being permanently overwhelmed by negative emotions, we learn ways to handle them, and thereby become stronger.

Instructions

1. *Find a place where you won't be interrupted for fifteen to thirty minutes.* A neutral place, such as a table placed in the corner of the room, works well.

2. *Write continuously for fifteen to thirty minutes for four or five consecutive days.* Pennebaker's original instructions are:

> I want you to write continuously about the most upsetting or traumatic experience of your entire life. Don't worry about grammar, spelling, or sentence structure. In your writing, I want you to discuss your deepest thoughts *and feelings* [italics added] about the experience. You can write about anything you want. But whatever you choose, it should be something that has affected you very deeply. Ideally, it should be something you have not talked about with others in detail. It is critical, however, that you let yourself go and touch those deepest emotions and thoughts that you have. In other words, write about what happened and how you felt about it, and how you feel about it now. Finally, you can write on different traumas during each session or the same one over the entire [period]. Your choice of trauma for each session is entirely up to you.

3. *Although it is usually beneficial, it isn't necessary to write about the most traumatic event of your life.* If a topic makes you overly distraught, ease up. Approach it gradually or try a different topic. In other words, you control the topic to explore and the pace.

4. *Write especially about topics that you dwell on and/or you would like to talk about but are embarrassed.* Write mostly about your feelings. Avoid wishful thinking (e.g., I wish he weren't dead; I'd like to get even), which is a way to avoid the underlying feelings. Instead, focus on your feelings and what they mean.

5. *Remember to write continuously for fifteen to thirty minutes.* If you run out of words, repeat yourself.

6. *Write just for yourself.* If you worry about someone reading it, you may not write what you honestly feel. (You might need to take special precautions to ensure that others do not read your journal.)

7. *Expect sadness immediately afterward.* This usually dissipates within an hour or, rarely, within a day or two. Most people then feel relief/contentment for up to six months afterward.

8. *Balance writing with action.* Don't let writing be a method of avoidance. Writing is not a substitute for remedial action. For example, you'll probably still need to tell others if they hurt your feelings and you want them to stop. Don't merely complain, which is a way to keep things the same and avoid action.

9. *Look ahead after discharging and analyzing your traumas.* Don't stay in a wallowing stage. As a rule, expressing and processing difficult experiences will help you to replay them less.

10. *This is not a substitute for therapy for intractable problems.* If writing is unduly disturbing, or you continue to feel distressed after the four days of writing, consider talking to a mental health professional. Like a good coach, a skilled mental health professional can facilitate the healing process by providing a supportive climate, helping to establish a reasonable pace, and teaching needed skills. For example, trauma specialists can help you to process difficult traumatic memories using a variety of skills, including eye move-

ment desensitization and reprocessing (EMDR), dream management, or prolonged exposure. Sometimes expressive art therapists can be very helpful. For example, a person who finds it difficult to talk about feelings might be able to draw or paint the feelings. It may feel more comfortable to talk about the feelings in the artistic creation.

Time Tripping

This imagery exercise is a very effective way to heal past wounds with compassion. You might start by identifying a difficult time in your past. Perhaps you felt diminished, disrespected, unprotected, or hurt. Or you might identify a present situation that triggers intense anger. Calmly try to pinpoint the feelings underneath your anger. Then trace back to a time in your life when you first felt such feelings (or go back as far as possible to find a situation where you felt these feelings). For example, let's say you feel intensely angry when your computer malfunctions or you don't know how to operate it efficiently. Underneath your anger you might be feeling helpless, weak, or alone. You might remember a time early in life when you felt helpless, small, and abandoned. Time tripping enables you to return to this time—from the perspective of greater wisdom, experience, and compassion—and modify the emotional content of the memory, replacing the painful feelings with supportive, soothing feelings. In effect, you neutralize the painful feelings with compassion so that the memory no longer interferes with your present life.

Instructions

1. Think of a difficult time back in the past when you felt alone, unprotected, or unassisted. Perhaps you were mistreated, frustrated, or interfered with. Call the person experiencing these feelings your Younger Self.

2. Relax your body. Take two easy, deep breaths, using your calming word or phrase as you breath in and as you breathe out.

3. Now imagine your present self, in possession of greater wisdom, experience, and compassion. Call this person your Wiser Self.

4. Imagine that this Wiser Self enters a time machine that takes you back to that painful time. The Wiser Self emerges from the time machine and sees the Younger Self. The Wiser and Younger Selves make eye contact. There seems to be a genuine affinity and trust between the two selves.

5. Perhaps the Wiser Self knows instinctively what is needed. Perhaps the Wiser Self asks the Younger Self what is troubling him/her, and listens compassionately and patiently as the Younger Self expresses the disappointment, hurt, fear, and/or abandonment. And the Wiser Self asks what is needed and how those needs can be met. And the Wiser Self provides for those needs, perhaps just being present with soothing, protective love. Perhaps a loving touch or embrace, or an affectionate look. Perhaps words of encouragement or advice (e.g., "You're just a child. You're doing well. You're loved and worthwhile. I know you'll make it."). Perhaps the Wiser Self moves close and provides physical protection or help talking back to an offender. Together they figure out what is needed and this time provide for those needs so that the pain is healed and the anger is released.

6. Perhaps the Wiser Self gives the Younger Self a token, a symbol of love and support to keep with him/her. Perhaps the Younger Self returns with the Wiser Self, back to the future, where the Younger Self is safe, secure, and content.

7. And now you are in the present, and you feel love, security, good cheer, and peace—and you meet all challenges with these feelings.

Drill

During the course of the day, try to simply describe what you are feeling. Say at least once, "I feel . . . (content, sad, frustrated, etc.)."

Reflections

How poor are they that have not patience; what wound did ever heal but by degrees!

(William Shakespeare, *Othello*)

Give sorrow words: The grief that does not speak whispers the o'erfraught heart, and bids it break.

(William Shakespeare, *Macbeth*)

Is life fair? NO! Life isn't fair. We are all at risk. We must choose how we will respond to pain.

(Anonymous)

To be wronged or robbed is nothing unless you continue to remember it.

(Confucius)

Suggested Activities

1. In your journal, write about your most upsetting life experiences over a four-day period. Follow the instructions in the "Confiding Hidden Wounds" section.
2. Do the "Time Tripping" exercise to heal a wound from the past. Describe the experience in your journal. (Writing about an exercise reinforces the benefits.)

9

Maintaining Equilibrium

If you're not meeting your most basic needs, you won't be of much use to yourself or anybody else.

—Anonymous

In Chapters 3 through 8 you have learned the foundational anger management skills. The skills in this chapter will help you maintain a calmer, more peaceful existence—reinforcing the habit of internal repose and well-being. The central assumption of this chapter is that keeping life more pleasant and balanced reduces the likelihood of overreacting.

Sound Body, Sound Mind

To remain in our very best emotional state requires that the body be optimally healthy. It is difficult to apportion the benefit to sound mental health contributed by sound physical health practices, but evidence indicates that one can't expect to feel one's best mentally without minding the body. We will discuss some important lifestyle considerations. If you are not presently following these recommendations, we recommend starting them very gradually, only making changes that you can follow for life.

Sleep Practices

Given the connection between fear and anger, it is indeed wise to remember that "fatigue makes cowards of us all." Insufficient rest has been linked to unhappiness and degraded mental health in numerous studies. Sometimes waking up "on the wrong side of the bed" is just a reflection of waking up insufficiently rested. Sleep deprivation has been associated with elevated stress hormones and blood sugars the following day. There is an emerging consensus among sleep researchers that adults require *at least* eight hours of sleep per night in order to feel and function at their best. At the turn of the twentieth century American adults averaged more than nine hours of sleep per night. In today's twenty-four-hour society, however, adults average less than seven hours per night. Even small increases in the amount of sleep per night seem to pay off in better functioning and mood states.

Regularity is a second important factor. With age, sleep cycles in the brain become more fragile and require consistent sleep and awakening cues to remain regular. The ideal is to retire and awake at regular times throughout the week. However, many people stay up later on the weekends and/or try to make up for their weekly sleep debt by sleeping in on the weekends. If one stays up a few hours later on Friday and Saturday, it may be difficult to fall asleep at the normal time on Sunday night. Insomnia is sometimes rooted in such maladaptive sleep practices. Try to keep the hours of retiring and awakening as consistent as possible, varying no more than one hour from night to night, and preferably less.

Shiftwork can exact a physical and mental toll. If it is necessary to engage in it, try to stay on a shift for as many weeks as possible in order to allow the body to adjust to the change. Also, try shifting from earlier to later shifts, which seems easier for the body to adjust to.

Sleep Tips

• Reserve the bedroom for sleeping and sex. Remove phones and televisions. Don't pay bills or work there. These can cause the bedroom to be associated with mental stimulation.

• Reduce light and noise. Early morning light coming through the window, light from a clock, or noise can disrupt sleep even if people are not aware of these. Noise can be masked by "white noise," such as a fan or a soothing noise box.

• Limit bedtime snacks to light carbohydrate and/or low-fat dairy snacks (e.g., warm milk, crackers and cheese, yogurt, bread). Don't eat a big meal within several hours of retiring.

• Avoid stimulants, such as caffeine, for at least seven to ten hours before bedtime. Alcohol also disrupts sleep.

• Either nap regularly (60 percent of adults seem to benefit from an early afternoon nap) or avoid naps altogether (to consolidate sleep if you are having difficulty sleeping at night).

• Try exercising several hours before going to bed (many find just before dinner to be helpful in reducing arousal).

• Try progressive muscle relaxation just before sleeping. (See Chapter 3.)

Eating Practices

Untold monies have been spent to develop dietary guidelines for American adults. If followed, these guidelines can reduce cardiovascular disease, cancer, diabetes, depression, and other stress-related diseases. They are not difficult or expensive to follow, yet less than 10 percent of adults do so, as obesity continues to increase.

Obsessed with losing weight, many adults try to *avoid* eating. As hunger mounts, they often turn to calorie-dense fast or processed foods. We suggest a plan where you concentrate on *eating* nourishing and satisfying foods. Focus on eating what you need to feel and function well and you won't need to fill up on unwise food choices.

If you visualize a plate where meat products comprise less than one fourth of the plate and plant foods fill the rest of the plate, then you have a pretty good idea of the dietary guidelines, which include the following:

• *Get most of your calories from plant foods.* Fruits, vegetables, and cereals/grains contain fiber, which tends to reduce and stabilize blood sugars and fats. They also provide many essential vitamins and minerals. Simply adding servings of fruits and vegetables to the diet has been shown to reduce weight and blood pressure. Eating a variety of plant foods will tend to neutralize the few naturally occurring plant foods that tend to raise blood sugar.

• *Reduce meats, which contain saturated fats and cholesterol, to about 6 ounces daily.* Use mainly lean meats, poultry without skin, fish, or meat alternates such as dry beans, peas, and nuts.

• *Reduce fats, sugar, salt, processed foods, caffeine, and alcohol.* Replacing processed foods with fresh or frozen foods eliminates much fat, salt, and sugar.

• *Take adequate calcium.* Adults require more than 1,000 milligrams per day. A glass of milk or fortified orange juice contains 300 milligrams. Broccoli, tofu, and various dark green vegetables also are good sources of calcium.

Other useful guidelines can help to stabilize the mood, control weight, and improve health generally.

• *Keep blood sugar steady throughout the day.* This can be done by eating breakfast, not skipping meals, and eating smaller, more frequent meals (a meal can be a mid-morning yogurt, or a mid-afternoon half-sandwich or fruit). Avoid concentrated sweets, which can cause a fatiguing drop in blood sugar after an initial blood sugar spike. Caffeine and alcohol can also affect blood sugar levels.

• *Drink lots of water.* Too little can lead to feelings of hunger, fatigue, and dehydration; it can also lead to fluid and fat retention. About eight glasses of water per day is recommended.

- *Eat sufficient calories each day.* Even modest reductions in calories can leave one feeling irritable. The average adult requires at least 2,000 calories per day to maintain weight; consuming fewer than 1,200 calories per day makes it unlikely that you'll be getting sufficient nutrients to sustain health. If you are trying to lose weight, aim to lose no more than about 1 pound per week. (If you exercise, this might translate into eating only about 250 calories less per day, the amount in a candy bar or half a cup of ice cream.) Severe caloric reduction runs the risk of slowing the body's metabolic rate and increasing aggressive tendencies. As an activity, make an eating plan for two weeks. List everything you plan to eat and drink for all meals and snacks, including water. Then check it against the dietary guidelines in Appendix A.

Gentle Physical Conditioning

Moderate, regular exercise is remarkably effective for improving mental and physical health. It measurably reduces muscle tension and other stress symptoms without the side effects of medication. It improves self-esteem, lowers blood pressure, slows resting breathing and heart rates, increases energy levels and stamina, improves the quality of sleep,[1] promotes weight loss, strengthens the immune system, reduces PMS symptoms, and reduces anxiety and depression. Although many people assume they are too busy to exercise, managers and students who exercise regularly have been found to accomplish more than those who did not. If life is a marathon rather than a sprint, then exercise is an investment that pays off in more energy and sharper functioning.

Some people think they are too old or out of shape to exercise. These, however, are the people who show the greatest benefit from starting a gentle program of exercise.

In terms of stress and anger, exercise also provides a natural outlet for the energy of arousal, leaving us more relaxed and refreshed. I think of my psychology professor at West Point, who said that he always felt very relaxed after football practice when he was in college. All his aggression was left on the playing field. Exercise also affords a time for the mind to spin free, a mini-vacation from problems.

We emphasize moderate, regular exercise, such as taking a stroll. The best form of exercise leaves you feeling refreshed, not exhausted. If you enjoy doing it, you will be more likely to continue. The base of an exercise program is aerobic exercise. This is rhythmic, continuous exercise, such as walking, swimming, low-impact aerobics, jogging, biking, stair climbing, and some racket games. Strive for at least twenty minutes most days. To reduce stress and lose weight, daily aerobic exercise at a gentle pace is excellent—perhaps a daily thirty- or forty-minute walk. A gentle pace means you could talk to a friend. Build up gradually. You might start by walking up the street for five minutes, and take two weeks or more to progress to twenty minutes of walking. There is no rush to meet a goal. Any effort is beneficial, as long as you don't overdo it. Even a ten-minute energy walk, getting up from the desk to take a break from stress every hour or two, increases energy and improves the mood. Allow five to ten minutes to warm up and cool down. If you have any health problems or known medical risk factors (such as diabetes, heart disease, or high blood pressure) or if you are over forty years of age, get a physical examination first and discuss your exercise plans with your doctor.

Strength training (lifting weights, calisthenics, or similar activities) and flexibility exercises (e.g., yoga, stretching, tai chi) confer additional benefits. For example, gaining muscle mass causes body fat to be burned faster. Yoga can keep the joints flexible and slow the effects of aging. Programs might be offered in your area. However, these types of exercises can be learned from books and videos and don't necessarily require expensive equipment. For example, one could lift cans or other light weights in the home.

Pleasant Activities Scheduling

We are grateful to Dr. Peter Lewinsohn and his colleagues for developing the Pleasant Events Schedule.[2] Although we tend to feel balanced when we're doing both needed and pleasant activities, sometimes we fall into the habit of omitting pleasant activities from our lives. Perhaps they are given up during periods of great stress and pressure, or during very busy times when it seems like there is no time for pleasure. If we only do what is needed long enough, we might eventually forget what used to give us pleasure, or even assume that these events won't be fun anymore. Scheduling pleasant activities can restore balance. As we do things that are pleasant, we begin to feel happier and less distressed. Maintaining reasonable levels of pleasant activities also helps to prevent drops in mood, when we become more prone to anger.

The exercise that follows will both help you to discover (or rediscover) what is pleasant for you and to make a plan to do some of these things.

Step 1: Exhibit 9.1, the Pleasant Events Schedule, lists a wide range of activities. In column 1, check those activities that you enjoyed in the past. Then rate from 1 to 10 how pleasant each checked item was. A score of 1 reflects mild pleasure; a score of 10 reflects great pleasure. This rating goes in column 1 also, beside each check mark. For example, if you very much enjoyed being with happy people but didn't enjoy being with friends/relatives, your first two items would look like this:

  ✓ (8)   _____   1. Being with happy people

  _____   _____   2. Being with friends/relatives

Step 2: In column 2, place a check if you've done the event in the past thirty days.

Step 3: Circle the number of the events that you'd probably enjoy (when you're feeling good, on a good day).

Step 4: Notice if there are many items you've enjoyed in the past that you are not doing very often (compare the first and second columns).

Step 5: Using the completed Pleasant Events Schedule for ideas, make a list of the twenty-five activities that you feel you'd enjoy most.

Exhibit 9.1 Pleasant Events Schedule

I. Social Interactions. These events occur with others. They tend to make us feel accepted, appreciated, liked, understood, etc.*

Column 1 Column 2

____	____	1. Being with happy people
____	____	2. Being with friends/relatives
____	____	3. Thinking about people I like
____	____	4. Planning an activity with people I care for
____	____	5. Meeting someone new of the same sex
____	____	6. Meeting someone new of the opposite sex
____	____	7. Going to a club, tavern, etc.
____	____	8. Being at celebrations (birthdays, weddings, baptisms, parties, family get-togethers, etc.)
____	____	9. Meeting a friend for lunch or a drink
____	____	10. Talking openly and honestly (e.g., about your hopes, your fears, what interests you, what makes you laugh, what saddens you)
____	____	11. Expressing true affection (verbal or physical)
____	____	12. Showing interest in others
____	____	13. Noticing successes and strengths in family and friends
____	____	14. Dating, courting (this one is for married people, too)
____	____	15. Having a lively conversation
____	____	16. Inviting friends over
____	____	17. Stopping in to visit friends
____	____	18. Calling up someone I enjoy talking to
____	____	19. Apologizing
____	____	20. Smiling at people
____	____	21. Calmly talking over problems with people I live with
____	____	22. Giving compliments, back pats, or praise
____	____	23. Good natured teasing/bantering
____	____	24. Amusing people or making them laugh
____	____	25. Playing with children
____	____	26. Others: _____

*You might feel that an activity belongs in another group. The grouping is not important.

II. Activities that make us feel capable, loving, useful, strong, or adequate.

Column 1   Column 2

____ ____	1.	Starting a challenging job or doing a job well
____ ____	2.	Learning something new (e.g., fixing leaks, new hobby, new language)
____ ____	3.	Helping someone (counseling, advising, listening)
____ ____	4.	Contributing to religious, charitable, or other groups
____ ____	5.	Driving skillfully
____ ____	6.	Expressing myself clearly (out loud or in writing)
____ ____	7.	Repairing something (sewing, fixing a car or bike, etc.)
____ ____	8.	Solving a problem or puzzle
____ ____	9.	Exercising
____ ____	10.	Thinking
____ ____	11.	Going to a meeting (convention, business, civic)
____ ____	12.	Visiting the ill, homebound, or troubled
____ ____	13.	Telling a child a story
____ ____	14.	Writing a card, note, or letter
____ ____	15.	Improving my appearance (e.g., seeking medical or dental help, improving my diet, going to a barber or beautician)
____ ____	16.	Planning/budgeting time
____ ____	17.	Discussing political issues
____ ____	18.	Doing volunteer work, community service, etc.
____ ____	19.	Planning a budget
____ ____	20.	Protesting injustice, protecting someone, stopping fraud or abuse
____ ____	21.	Being honest, moral, etc.
____ ____	22.	Correcting mistakes
____ ____	23.	Organizing a party
____ ____	24.	Others: _____

III. Intrinsically Pleasant Activities

____ ____	1.	Laughing
____ ____	2.	Relaxing, having peace and quiet
____ ____	3.	Having a good meal

Exhibit 9.1 (Continued)

Column 1   Column 2

_____ _____ 4. A hobby (e.g., cooking, fishing, woodworking, photography, acting, gardening, collecting things)

_____ _____ 5. Listening to good music

_____ _____ 6. Seeing beautiful scenery

_____ _____ 7. Going to bed early, sleeping soundly, and awakening early

_____ _____ 8. Wearing attractive clothes

_____ _____ 9. Wearing comfortable clothes

_____ _____ 10. Going to a concert, opera, ballet, or play

_____ _____ 11. Playing sports (e.g., tennis, softball, racquetball, golf, horseshoes)

_____ _____ 12. Trips or vacations

_____ _____ 13. Shopping/buying something I like for myself

_____ _____ 14. Being outdoors (e.g., beach, country, mountains, kicking leaves, walking in the sand, floating in lakes)

_____ _____ 15. Doing artwork (e.g., painting, sculpture, drawing)

_____ _____ 16. Reading sacred works

_____ _____ 17. Beautifying my home (redecorating, cleaning, yardwork, etc.)

_____ _____ 18. Going to a sports event

_____ _____ 19. Reading (novels, poems, magazines, newspapers, etc.)

_____ _____ 20. Going to a lecture

_____ _____ 21. Going for a drive

_____ _____ 22. Sitting in the sun

_____ _____ 23. Visiting a museum

_____ _____ 24. Playing or singing music

_____ _____ 25. Boating

_____ _____ 26. Pleasing my family, friends, employer

_____ _____ 27. Thinking about something good in the future

_____ _____ 28. Watching TV

_____ _____ 29. Camping, hunting

_____ _____ 30. Grooming myself (e.g., bathing, combing hair, shaving)

Column 1   Column 2

____	____	31. Writing in my diary/journal
____	____	32. Taking a bike ride, hiking, or walking
____	____	33. Being with animals
____	____	34. Watching people
____	____	35. Taking a nap
____	____	36. Listening to nature sounds
____	____	37. Getting or giving a backrub
____	____	38. Watching a storm, clouds, the sky, etc.
____	____	39. Having spare time
____	____	40. Daydreaming
____	____	41. Feeling the presence of a Higher Power in my life. Praying, worshiping, etc.
____	____	42. Smelling a flower
____	____	43. Talking about old times or special interests
____	____	44. Going to auctions, garage sales, etc.
____	____	45. Traveling
____	____	46. Others: _____

Step 6: Make a written plan to do more pleasant activities. You might start with the simpler activities that you are most likely to enjoy. Do as many pleasant events as you reasonably can. We suggest doing at least one each day, perhaps more on weekends. *Write* your plan on a calendar and carry out this written plan for at least two weeks. Each time you do an activity, rate it on a 1 to 5 scale for pleasure (5 being highly enjoyable). This tests the idea that *nothing* is enjoyable. Later, you can replace less enjoyable activities with others. Don't be surprised if some of your old favorites are not so enjoyable at first, especially if your mood is low. Try some other activities, and then gradually try your old favorites as your mood lifts.

Some Additional Tips

• Tune into the physical world. Pay less attention to your thoughts. Feel the wind or the soap suds as you wash the car. See and hear.

• Before doing an event, set yourself up to enjoy it. Identify three things you will enjoy about it. Say "I will enjoy _____ (the sunshine, the breeze, talking with my brother Bill, etc.)." Relax and imagine yourself enjoying each aspect of the event as you repeat each statement.

• Ask yourself, "What will I do to make the activity enjoyable?" Sometimes the answer is to just relax and enjoy it, without trying to control it.

• If you are concerned that you might not enjoy some activity that you'd like to try, try breaking it up into steps. Think small, so you can be satisfied in reaching your goal. For example, start by only cleaning the house for ten minutes, then stop. Then reward yourself with a "Good job!" pat on the back.

• Check your schedule for balance. Can you spread out the "need to's" to make room for some "want to's"?

• Time is limited, so use it wisely. You needn't do activities you don't like just because they're convenient.

Keeping an Anger Journal

If you haven't already started, try writing about your anger in a daily anger journal. Describe the event that triggered your anger. Then describe the full range of feelings. Remember, journaling conveys the message that your feelings are acceptable and gives you a constructive way to understand and process those feelings. Writing slows things down. You get a chance to explore all the feelings below the anger. Often your confusing, complex feelings will begin to make sense, and you'll feel better after expressing and discharging them in a way that hurts no one. You might find yourself better able to discuss and resolve those feelings with others. If anger arises like steam in a pressure cooker, a journal can serve as a release valve for the rising pressure—a preventive measure to address hurts before you explode. Don't just focus on the negative feelings. You might also record what you feel good about or explore other ways to view the offense.

A journal can be a simple loose-leaf notebook that no one besides you sees. Generally, write for about thirty minutes each day, in a neutral place that you don't want to be associated with arousal. For example, you might choose a chair in a corner, rather than the bedroom or the kitchen table.

Pleasant Imagery Recall

This activity is extremely pleasant in its own right. It is also a very nice way to end a journaling session. Angry people typically recall memories with irritation, seeming to forget pleasant aspects of their lives or taking limited pleasure from their memories. This activity will challenge you to reexperience pleasant memories from your past, vividly and in great detail, without letting anger or other negative feelings ruin the pleasure of the activity. An advantage of this exercise is that it draws from material that is already stored in memory, so it promotes the feeling of constructive power to realize that we each have within us the capacity to lift our own spirits. Try it separately at first. Then try it after you make a journal entry as a way to realize that you can control your feelings. That is, you can acknowledge anger or hurts, express the feelings, and then end up feeling good again.

Pleasant Imagery Recall Instructions

In this exercise, you will recall in vivid detail a very pleasant experience from your life. If you recall it in sufficient detail, your brain and body will experience reactions that are very similar to those that you actually experienced during the pleasant experience. Should you at any time experience negative thoughts that could pull you out of the pleasant experience (e.g., you remember something negative that happened later), firmly and calmly think, "Stop. I won't allow those negative thoughts in to ruin this experience." Then return to recalling the pleasant memory. If you prefer, put the instructions on an audiotape or have someone read them to you.

1. To begin, sit or lie down in a very comfortable place. You might choose a soft chair, a bed, a sofa, or the floor.

2. Completely relax your body. Passively release tension. Take two easy, deep breaths, saying your calming word or phrase as you breathe in and as you breathe out. Then breathe so that only your abdomen moves, normally, quietly, gently. Release and relax as your mind becomes clear and calm.

3. Sitting or lying now in your very safe place, perhaps you remember a time in your life when you felt very safe and protected. And you feel that way now . . . very safe . . . very protected.

4. Imagine that your closed eyelids are like a big blank, white screen. From your relaxed vantage point, you see several of your happiest, most pleasant memories floating across the screen. When you have identified two or three of your most happy memories, select one that is particularly pleasant.

5. Begin to recall that pleasant event in great detail. First, recall all the visual aspects of the memory. Slowly scan the setting so that you see all the details in that scene . . . things that were far away, close, and all in between. Things that were over you and below you. Recall shades, textures, colors. (Pause) And you can vividly recall sounds in that image, as well . . . soft sounds, louder sounds, all sounds. (Pause). And you recall tactile sensations . . . what your body felt. Perhaps the temperature of the air or things that were touching you. (Pause) And you perhaps recall what the air smelled like . . . and perhaps you remember tastes. (Pause). Because this was such a pleasant memory, you can remember the particulars in vivid detail. Take a moment to recall even more of these details. (Pause).

And you now remember what you were feeling when you experienced that moment. Let your body feel those feelings, those emotions. Let your relaxed face express those feelings . . . whether it be through a smile or perhaps an expression of serenity. Allow yourself to simply experience those feelings for a few more moments.

6. And now let your attention return to the present, as you feel relaxed, alert, and pleasant.

Try repeating this imagery for other pleasant life experiences. You might find that you'll access memories you thought were long forgotten—ranging from very pleasant to calm, simple moments (such as lying under a tree). We recommend that you record the details of the memories in your journal. Doing so makes the memories even more vivid and accessible. Soon you will have a record of many pleasant moments. Rereading the record can be a great source of comfort during stressful times.

Time Management and Getting Organized

Technological advances were supposed to make life easier. Instead, they have increased the complexities and expectations of modern living, leaving many people feeling overwhelmed, exhausted, and irritable. Increasingly, time management has become a vital survival skill. But time management is more than learning to juggle multiple demands efficiently. *Too many angry, driven people are efficient but miserable—rich in achievements but impoverished in joy and health. Wise time management involves taking the time to develop a peaceful and balanced life plan, fight overload, and set reasonable expectations.*

There are several antidotes to the exhaustion, or burnout, that afflicts so many people today. One is to take vacations that are long enough to refresh. Americans are taking considerably less vacation time than they did thirty years ago. This is unfortunate, since taking regular vacations is associated with better health. A second antidote is to develop and live by a plan that balances work, love, and play. The "want to's" of life are just as essential to overall well-being as the "need to's" because the former promote growth, satisfaction, joy, and emotional well-being. This is not to diminish the importance of "need to's." There is nothing wrong with well-defined career goals that promote prosperity. The strategy presented here, however, will challenge you to also meet your essential emotional, physical, and spiritual needs, so that you are more likely to achieve your professional goals without burning out and losing the "*joie de vivre*." Get some sheets of paper and be prepared to write.

Step 1: *Life Goals*. Finish the following sentence stems. Write as quickly as you can. Do not worry about whether what you write is doable or makes sense. Just write quickly.

- My personal definition of success is . . . (Try to think beyond the material. Several studies have shown that people whose central goals are solely financial tend to have poorer mental health.)
- If I were to live more fully functioning and happily, I would be more _____ and less _____. (For this one, indicate personal traits, e.g., more patient and less irritable.)
- My life overall would be just about ideal/complete if I were to . . . (Imagine you were taking a video of yourself. What would you see yourself doing?)
- My retirement goals are . . .
- My goals for ten years from now are . . .
- My goals for five years from now are . . .
- My goals for one year from now are . . .
- If someone looking into a crystal ball were to tell me that I had only six months to live, I would do the following: _____

Step 2: *Balance Check*. You have just made a substantial list of goals that are important to you. Now you'll check your goals for balance. Goals typically fall under one or more of the following categories:

1. *Physical health* (weight, fitness, rest, eating, medical care)
2. *Personal growth* (character/spiritual development, personality traits, emotional health)
3. *Relationships* (family, friends, groups)
4. *Recreation* (entertainment, hobbies, travel, reading)
5. *Professional* (career or educational)
6. *Possessions* (things you'd like to acquire, earnings)

Beside each response to the sentence stems in Step 1, place a 1, 2, 3, 4, 5, and/or a 6 according to the six categories above. When you finish this step, pause. What do you notice? Are your goals balanced? Make any desired adjustments.

Step 3: *Backward Planning.* There is peace in preparation, in having a sound written plan to refer to during times of distraction and distress. In this step, translate your general life goals into more specific goals that are achievable. Start by making a Five-Year Goals sheet as illustrated in Table 9.1.

Considering all your life goals, list several goals under each of the six categories listed in Step 2. Try to make each goal as specific and measurable as possible. For example, instead of the vague physical health goal of "improve appearance," you might write "lose 1 inch off waistline." Instead of "improve personal relationships," you might write "spend fifteen minutes of uninterrupted time with my daughter each day." In the second column, list specific steps that will enable you to reach each goal. For example, a way to lose 1 inch from the waistline might be to walk for thirty minutes six days a week. In the third column, specify when you will begin to work on each goal. In the fourth column, describe how you will measure/observe the successful achievement of each goal (e.g., achieve waist measurement of 30 inches). The last column is completed after the five-year time period.

Table 9.1 Five-Year Goals

for Period _____ 20___ to _____ 20___

(month/year)   *(month/year)*

Goals	What I'll Do to Reach Goals	Starting Date	How I'll Know I Reached Goals	How I Did (evaluate at end of period)

Continue the backward planning process by completing a One-Year Goals sheet next. Make a separate sheet for your goals for the coming year, following the same procedures as for the Five-Year Goals sheet.

Step 4: *Monthly Planning.* Next, complete a monthly calendar for the upcoming month. What will you do each day to bring you closer to your five- and one-year goals? Anticipate and record here major events coming up during the month, such as medical or professional appointments, work tasks, and recreational dates. You might wish to make or buy a monthly planner to continue planning for each month.

Step 5: *Weekly Planning.* Plan a typical week, using the form in Table 9.2.

Table 9.2 Typical Weekly Work and Recreation Schedule

Hours	Sunday	Monday	Tuesday	Wednesday	Thursday	Friday	Saturday
6–7 A.M.							
7–8							
8–9							
etc.							

It is wise to start by blocking out some of the essentials (such as sleep, eating, exercise, pleasant activities) before you block out other demands (commuting, work, meetings). Remember, life is a marathon. You'll run farther and accomplish more if you are conditioned, rested, and nourished. You'll probably want to include perhaps an hour of time at week's beginning to plan the week.

Pause here for a moment. Have you allowed time each day for emotional, spiritual, and physical nourishment? If not, you will probably not give your best to yourself, others, or your tasks. Is there ample time allocated to accomplish your monthly goals? If overloading is evident, what would happen if you softened expectations or spread out some of your goals? Remember, you can do almost anything you choose to do, but you can't do everything, and you can't do it all at once. Do what you can, and then be satisfied, since no one can do more than that.

Step 6:   *Daily "To Do" List.* Make a single list of things you choose to do for the upcoming day, by their priority. Do the highest priority items first. Try to make a list with reasonable expectations, allowing sufficient time to accomplish each item. If you don't get to all the items, place the unfinished items on tomorrow's "to do" list, again listed by priority. You might wish to make a "to do" list at least an hour or two before retiring and review it at the start of the next day. It is also suggested that you keep all your planning sheets together, perhaps in a single notebook, with your daily "to do" list first, where you can refer to it often.

Time Management Tips

• Plan to arrive at a destination at least ten minutes early. If the activity is important or if delays are likely (traffic, etc.), plan to arrive earlier.

• Bring a book or something else to do, so that you can stay calm if you are kept waiting.

• Stay on task. Once you have a balanced plan, work efficiently so that you will have time to recreate. Don't waste time.

• Have a contingency plan. Anticipate glitches so that you can stay calm. Make copies of important papers and store them in a different place from the original. Have coins in the car for parking meters. Have a spare key in your wallet in case you lock yourself out of the car. Leave a spare house key with neighbors or safely hidden outside the house.

• Organize. Develop a retrieval system for important information. Get a file cabinet with folders for taxes, medical information, budget, insurance papers, assets (and where they are located in case of emergency), and other important papers. Get rid of clutter—needless papers, clothes you haven't worn in a year, etc. Store clothes and tools so that you can put your hands on them. Keep a notebook of lists so that you don't have to hunt for them. Lists could include birthdays, gifts to buy and sizes, addresses and phone numbers, things you'd like to buy for fun, or favorite books and movies.

Drills

• Eat more slowly. Consciously enjoy each bite.
• Practice arriving ten minutes early to social events. Enjoy the feeling of watching people enter.
• Cause yourself to take extra steps. (Walk instead of taking the elevator, park farther away, etc.)

- Take care to notice pleasant scenery: flowers, sky, grass, etc.
- Walk and drive slower. Notice the scenery.
- Smile pleasantly at people passing by.
- Look closely at a flower or a single leaf.
- Recall pleasant memories for ten minutes. Record them in your journal.

Reflections

Unless each day can be looked back upon by an individual as one in which he has had some fun, some joy, some real satisfaction, that day is a loss.

(Dwight D. Eisenhower)

When was the last time you really listened to raindrops; looked at the face of your spouse, child, or mother; looked at your own face in a moment of peace?

(Anonymous)

Suggested Activities

1. Make a written, two-week plan to take care of your body. Include sufficient, regular sleep and exercise, and daily meal plans. Check your meal plan against the dietary guidelines in Appendix A. Try the plan for two weeks, make any needed adjustments, and continue following the plan.
2. Using your list of twenty-five favorite pleasant activities, make a two-week plan to enjoy at least one a day.
3. Complete the instructions in the "Time Management" section of this chapter. Make sure your monthly, weekly, and daily written plans first make provisions for your physical health and your pleasant activities.

10

Peace Within

No person can truly be at peace with himself if he does not live up to his moral capacity.

—Norman Cousins[1]

DAN WAS ARTICULATE, well groomed, handsome, and successful. He had an aura of earnest resolve and calm purpose. From outward appearances, he could have been a mental health professional or perhaps a clergyman. He wasn't. Dan was attending a court-ordered anger management class. Months before he had choked his beloved wife, from whom he was now separated. What circumstances had led to this outcome? For various reasons, Dan had begun using drugs. At one point his wife called the police because his anger was out of control. Dan said, "I'd resented her for humiliating me. This resentment brewed for a year. Finally, my anger erupted over a rather trivial disagreement. This is when I tried to choke her." This eruption and their subsequent separation became a wake-up call for Dan. He related, "In the many moments that I had to be alone and reflect, I came to realize that the situation was my own fault. My wife had become distant because I was getting out of control and dangerous while I was doing drugs. I forgave her—it wasn't really her fault. I resolved to get off drugs and become the person I know

I can be. I got help—private counseling from both a mental health professional and a pastoral counselor. I now worship regularly and found that has helped immensely. I got off drugs completely and stopped the other behaviors I'd been doing that were making me miserable—including the pornography and the affairs. I'm committed to spiritual growth and kindness. I am not pressing her to take me back, although that's what I desire. I am just showing her that I am genuinely changing. No excuses. I just try each day to be a better, more loving me. I hope she'll want to be with me again. It seems to be working . . . but if she doesn't, I'll still strive to be my best self—for my own inner happiness and peace of mind."

We human beings all sometimes do things that disappoint ourselves. We ask, what kind of a person would do such a thing? The answer is, "Not a very good one." An inner pain is created when we dislike what we are doing and what we are becoming, and this pain can be expressed as anger toward others. It is difficult to love someone who has hurt you—especially when that person is you. However, if we look honestly at ourselves, with great compassion, and find the love and resolve to replace unkind behaviors with constructive ones, inner peace can be restored. Anger can hide the pain, while keeping the inner pain as it is. An honest, loving look is required to identify the real source of the pain. These ideas are found in diverse cultures throughout history. For example, the Dalai Lama taught: "To be aware of a single shortcoming within oneself is more useful than to be aware of a thousand in somebody else."[2] Jesus taught: "And why beholdest thou the mote that is in thy brother's eye, but considerest not the beam that is in thine own eye?" (Matt. 7:3) We are far less likely to condemn others for their weaknesses once we have taken responsibility to acknowledge and correct our own. Perhaps we gain compassion as we realize how difficult self-mastery is.

Can each person achieve inner peace? Mother Teresa was once asked by a reporter what it was like to be a living saint. She replied, "You have to be holy in your position as you are, and I have to be holy in the position that God has put me. So it is nothing extraordinary to be holy. Holiness is not the luxury of the few. Holiness is a simple duty for you and for me. We have been created for that."[3] Thus, one can be holy as a teacher, parent, politician, or trash collector. *Holy* is an interesting word. It derives from the same root as *health* and *whole*, and means integrity—no discrepancy between one's behavior and one's values. When our behaviors accord with our best ideals, then we feel greater peace and happiness. In fact, the Greek word for happiness, *eudaimonia*, literally means "good soul." So the antidote to this kind of spiritual pain is to first change ourselves, gaining greater inner peace so that the pain doesn't erupt as anger. Inner happiness and peace derive in large part from living up to our moral potential. As we do, we begin to develop an intact sense of self, an inner confidence and security. Rogers writes: "It's not the honors and the prizes and the fancy outsides of life which ultimately nourish our souls. It's the knowing that we can be trusted, that we never have to fear the truth, that the bedrock of our very being is good stuff. That's what makes growing humanity the most potentially glorious enterprise on earth."[4]

While holy living is essential to inner peace and mental health, this does not imply that one must be perfectly holy to feel at peace. It does imply that we are on course and trying our best, since that is all anyone can do. Since no one is perfect, we can hope for a "clear but forgiving interior voice to guide" us.[5]

The Loving, Fearless, Searching, and Honest Moral Inventory

This activity is patterned after the Moral Inventory of Alcoholics Anonymous. When grocers inventory their shelves, they simply count what is there without judging. This counting enables them to rationally make needed adjustments. Likewise, when we inventory our own strengths and weaknesses, we can simply notice what is there without judging the core self.

The inventory process is *honest*. Without truth, we cannot trust ourselves, nor will anyone else. It is *fearless* and *searching* because loving acceptance of our fallible selves empowers us to see all aspects of ourselves clearly. It is a *moral* inventory, not an *immoral* inventory, because both strengths and weaknesses are identified.

Since all people are different and imperfect, it is of little value to compare your present development to that of others or to be discouraged because you are not further along. What is useful is to be honestly aware of your present state, and satisfied that you are moving in a desired direction and at a sustainable pace.

The process of developing inner peace follows three steps:

1. Identify present strengths. Seeing strengths alongside weaknesses helps to put the shortcomings in perspective. It is motivating to realize that some strengths and much potential already exist.
2. Identify present weaknesses. In a loving and forgiving way, try to acknowledge them so that you can improve upon them.
3. Strengthen weak areas.

Step 1:   *Identify Present Moral Strengths.* Something is considered moral if it is in the long-term best interest of humanity, including yourself. Listed in Exhibit 10.1 are characteristics that are generally considered moral. Rate each characteristic according to the degree to which you have developed it. A rating of 10 means it is developed as much as is humanly possible. A rating of 0 means it is completely undeveloped; never demonstrated. Think of your ratings as a unique portrait. Perhaps some areas will shine quite brightly. Some areas will perhaps be undistinguished. And in some areas the light might not shine too much. Yet each portrait is uniquely valuable. This is not a competition; no one but you will see this, so relax and rate the areas as honestly as you can.

Step 2:   *Identify Present Moral Weaknesses.* Immoral conduct is considered to be that which is not in the long-term interest of humanity, including yourself. Generally, weaknesses would be considered the opposites of the strengths listed in Exhibit 10.1.

Take a few moments now to reflect upon this question: "What is presently disrupting my inner peace?"

- Are there any behaviors that are inconsiderate, unkind, self-indulgent, neglectful, or selfish? Am I using, exploiting, or manipulating others in any way? Do I lie, cheat, or steal in any way?

Exhibit 10.1 Identify Your Moral Strengths

Along the left are listed characteristics generally considered to be moral.

For each characteristic, or set of characteristics, circle the number on the scale that reflects the degree to which you have developed this characteristic in yourself.

Respectful
of others

Completely Undeveloped — Fully Developed

0 1 2 3 4 5 6 7 8 9 10

Respectful
of self

Completely Undeveloped — Fully Developed

0 1 2 3 4 5 6 7 8 9 10

Considerate,
thoughtful

Completely Undeveloped — Fully Developed

0 1 2 3 4 5 6 7 8 9 10

Caring,
affectionate

Completely Undeveloped — Fully Developed

0 1 2 3 4 5 6 7 8 9 10

Dependable,
responsible,
keeps word

Completely Undeveloped — Fully Developed

0 1 2 3 4 5 6 7 8 9 10

Fair

Completely Undeveloped — Fully Developed

0 1 2 3 4 5 6 7 8 9 10

Helpful

Completely Undeveloped — Fully Developed

0 1 2 3 4 5 6 7 8 9 10

Loyal,
trustworthy

Completely Undeveloped — Fully Developed

0 1 2 3 4 5 6 7 8 9 10

Honest
with self

Completely Undeveloped — Fully Developed

0 1 2 3 4 5 6 7 8 9 10

Exhibit 10.1 (Continued)

Honest with others

Completely Undeveloped — Fully Developed

0　1　2　3　4　5　6　7　8　9　10

Compassionate, empathic, tolerant of differences

Completely Undeveloped — Fully Developed

0　1　2　3　4　5　6　7　8　9　10

Patient, kind

Completely Undeveloped — Fully Developed

0　1　2　3　4　5　6　7　8　9　10

Humble, willing to admit faults

Completely Undeveloped — Fully Developed

0　1　2　3　4　5　6　7　8　9　10

Morally clean, chaste

Completely Undeveloped — Fully Developed

0　1　2　3　4　5　6　7　8　9　10

Faithful

Completely Undeveloped — Fully Developed

0　1　2　3　4　5　6　7　8　9　10

Friendly

Completely Undeveloped — Fully Developed

0　1　2　3　4　5　6　7　8　9　10

Forgiving

Completely Undeveloped — Fully Developed

0　1　2　3　4　5　6　7　8　9　10

Gentle

Completely Undeveloped — Fully Developed

0　1　2　3　4　5　6　7　8　9　10

Courteous

Completely Undeveloped — Fully Developed

0　1　2　3　4　5　6　7　8　9　10

	Completely Undeveloped									Fully Developed
Grateful, appreciative	0	1	2	3	4	5	6	7	8	9	10

	Completely Undeveloped									Fully Developed
Thrifty	0	1	2	3	4	5	6	7	8	9	10

	Completely Undeveloped									Fully Developed
Sharing	0	1	2	3	4	5	6	7	8	9	10

- Am I choosing any behaviors that are not in my own best interest because they are not loving, responsible, or uplifting?
- Am I clinging to anything that is illusory or unimportant—any habits that carry a high price tag?
- Are there any areas where I am choosing darkness rather than light?

Write about this in your journal, if you like, to help clarify your thoughts.

Step 3: *Strengthen Weak Areas.* Ask yourself:

- How would my life be different were I to strengthen the weaker areas?
- What could I do to change or grow? (Think of specific changes. What resources, if any, are needed to assist you in making these changes?)

Take one or two characteristics you would like to strengthen. Make a specific plan to follow for a few weeks. Then return to your inventory to evaluate progress and make further plans for improvement.

Please note that your portrait is a masterpiece in development. It is an ongoing process. Expect ascent to be difficult and that it will take time. Take responsibility to resolve guilt by acknowledging mis takes, making amends (acknowledge the hurt that was caused by your choices, apologize, restore losses as far as possible), and lovingly and optimistically committing to improve. Don't define yourself by previous mistakes. Each individual person is much more than his or her mistakes.

Drill

Start the day with the thought, "Today I will be as honest and decent as I can." Repeat throughout the week. Notice moral momentum building.

Reflections

The fault, dear Brutus, is not in our stars, but in ourselves.
(William Shakespeare, *Julius Caesar*)

Nothing brings peace but triumph of principles.
(Ralph Waldo Emerson)

You can't have a moral holiday and remain moral.
(Oswald Chambers)[6]

There is no debate possible when conscience speaks.
(Oswald Chambers)

There is only one thing that remains to us, that cannot be taken away: to act with courage and dignity and to stick to the ideals that give meaning to your life.
(Jawaharlal Nehru)

All is lovely outside my house and inside my house and myself.
(Winslow Homer)

Suggested Activity

Complete the Loving, Fearless, Searching, and Honest Moral Inventory (page 163). Take your time. Make and follow a plan for moral growth and inner peace.

11

Reducing Hostility

I will permit no man to narrow and degrade my soul by making me hate him.

—Booker T. Washington

Racial hatred would have little effect on one who has set his mind to do good for his fellowmen, black or white.

—George Washington Carver

HOSTILITY IS AN attitude of dislike and distrust toward other people. It assumes that others are bad at heart and will deliberately do something to hurt us. It usually promotes anger by putting us on the defensive, anticipating slights and offenses, and preparing us to do battle (or flee). Hostility wishes ill for other people. It has been associated with cardiovascular diseases and increased mortality from all causes, not to mention the damage it does to careers and relationships.

The person with a high level of hostility usually feels justified in having it. Certainly there are good reasons to acquire hostility. Consider how you might arrange the life of trusting children so that they would learn to dislike and distrust people.

First, we might have the parents lie, severely criticize and punish, or neglect the children. At the dinner table, the children might hear the parents talk cynically about other people, such as coworkers, or racial or ethnic groups. Growing up, the children may encounter "friends" who shun them or break confidences. As young adults, they may fall in love with people who are unfaithful, abusive, or who only love them for the money they earn. At work, they might have supervisors who only value productivity, never show interest in them as individuals, or don't promote fairly. The hostile view might become cemented when the individual finally loses hope and goes over to similarly bad behavior. For example, recall that near his death Stalin confided to Khrushchev that he trusted no one, not even himself.

Although children start out life with naive trust and liking, with maturity they learn that there are times when universal trust and liking are unwise. Certainly, ill will does exist in some people. As Satre said, "If the Jew did not exist, the anti-Semite would invent him."[1] Some people hate and have grown cold and inconsiderate. As Schweitzer said, some people may have blunted their essential kindness and become thoughtless and distracted by their selfish goals and fears. Thus, wisdom dictates that distrust be flexible and judicious, rather rare, and reserved for appropriate cases.

We recall a dialogue between Caine and Master Po in the television series "Kung Fu" that beautifully demonstrates the middle path. Caine asked how one maintains one's peace and composure when people in one's path are often hurtful. Master Po told him that the peace must come from within. First try to move around such people. If you cannot avoid them, then step back and see them as being in pain. View these people as imperfect rather than evil. Maintain compassion and understanding, yet remain disengaged from their harmful ways. The wise man neither permits abuse nor is hardened to suffering. If you must contend with the inevitable violence, do so with calmness, strength, and kindness, not a heart of destruction.

In other words, it is possible to take strong countermeasures, but without malice or hatred. Sometimes strong love for the offender can motivate us to stop him from behaving self-destructively.

In terms of its cumulative costs, hostility is not to our advantage. Hostility becomes a problem when we fixate on flaws (i.e., zero in on bad behaviors), then overgeneralize. We either say, "This person is *totally* that way," or "*All* of these people are like that." The question is: "To what degree do I generalize hostility and assume that people are mostly bad and desirous of deliberately hurting others?"

Sometimes the problem lies in our world view. If our lens on the world is colored by hostility, we might too readily assume that people are bad without scientifically challenging that assumption. In our experience, few people acknowledge that they are hostile. This is understandable because hostility is rarely an all-or-nothing condition, and because it seems so justified. So the better question is: "To what degree have I become hostile?" If we feel that we have become excessively hostile, then we can ask: "How might I prudently reduce my level of hostility? How might I increase my feelings of goodwill, liking, and trust of others?" There are many effective approaches.

Strategies to Reduce Hostility

1. Start by doing a cost–benefit analysis of hostility. Ronald Reagon's son said that his father couldn't imagine someone not liking him or wanting to do him harm. So he engaged people with a warmth that served him well throughout his political career. By contrast, Richard Nixon was politically derailed as a consequence of his hostility. Ask: "Is hostility serving me? Is it a problem in terms of its costs?"

2. Choose to reduce hostility. Like anger, hostility is a choice. We can choose to turn it down. Decide to like people and give people the benefit of the doubt more often. Approach people with a friendly attitude, assuming that they will respond in kind. Give off positive regard. Expect that people might respond with positive regard for you. Expect encounters to be enjoyable. If some are not, think, "That's okay. That's life."

3. Find evidence of goodness in people, which disputes the all-or-nothing distortion. Over the course of a week, seek at least ten evidences that people, though not perfect, often behave kindly, in ways that elevate humanity. For example:

- Raoul Wallenberg, Swedish diplomat, saved at least twenty thousand Hungarian Jews from Nazi death camps by issuing Swedish passports before dying in a Russian prison.
- A white man helped thousands of slaves to freedom through the Underground Railroad. When he died, four black men stopped the wagon carrying his coffin. In reverence, they carried the coffin on their backs up the hill to the grave site.
- At a University of Maryland sleepout, students sleeping on cardboard and concrete raised hunger awareness and $800 for the homeless.
- Over fifty thousand Germans have been identified who helped WWII Jews.[2]
- A brave Polish woman, Irene Gut Opdyke, hid twelve Jews in the basement of the Nazi major's home where she worked as a housekeeper during WWII. At night she smuggled food downstairs to the hiding Jews.[3]
- Albert Schweitzer, awarded the Nobel Peace Prize in 1952, sacrificed a comfortable life and promising career to devote himself to the practice of medicine in equatorial Africa. Once a crippled boy he had treated tried to help him carry luggage on a train. Thereafter, Schweitzer looked for people, rich or poor, to help.[4] Other Nobel Peace Prize recipients, including Mother Teresa, Martin Luther King, Jr., Doctors Without Borders, and the Dalai Lama, sacrificed personal comfort for noble causes.
- In *Sports Illustrated*,[5] Michael Silver described two famous friends: Joe Montana and Ronnie Lott. These Hall of Fame football players are quite different on the surface: white versus black, offense versus defense, country boy versus city kid. But they became confidants under difficult circumstances. Their families vacationed together, they cared for each other's kids, and they helped launch a children's television show. They describe their friendship as genuine, lasting a lifetime. If they were to wake up and find that everything had been taken away, they feel they'd

still be there for each other. Said Lott, "I feel Joe would be there for me, as I would for him."

- Viktor Frankl observed that while some concentration camp prisoners behaved like pigs, others chose to behave like saints, going around and serving their comrades.
- A professional football player drove one hundred miles to participate in a "Kids Day." He jumped into a rain-filled construction pit to rescue three drowning children, even though he could not swim. Although he managed to rescue one of the children, he himself drowned.
- Worldwide, the majority of lost wallets are returned.[6]
- Can you think of times when people were kind to you? How did it make you feel?
- Catch people doing acts of everyday kindness (cashiers, teachers, police officers, firefighters, little league coaches, someone holding a door or letting you merge in front of them on a crowded highway, your kids cleaning up for you without being asked).

4. Try to convince someone that a disliked person (a boss, a spouse, a coworker) is totally evil. Then try to convince the person that the disliked person is not all bad. This exercise tends to reinforce the idea that all good or all bad extremes rarely exist. Most people are somewhere in the middle.

5. Cultivate empathy and compassion. As Gulley states, empathy is "when somebody's crying but someone else is tasting the tears."[7] Try to understand the offender's viewpoint or perspective on the problem, their suffering, and why they might be behaving that way. Try to put yourself in the other person's shoes. Then show compassion, which is sorrow for another's suffering and the desire to help.

Ask yourself, "Why might someone do something like that? Have I looked at it from the other person's point of view?" Imagine other perspectives on the problem. Have deep, considerate feelings.

- Perhaps the curt waitress is harried or is having a bad day or trouble at home.

- Perhaps the inconsiderate driver is old, distracted, in a hurry for an important meeting, on the way to the hospital, etc.
- Perhaps an unruly child is afraid and unsettled by chaos at home or the anxiety of a caretaker.

Such compassion and restraint is beautifully illustrated in the following story related by Terry Dobson, who was then a student of aikido. (Aikido is a form a martial arts that teaches its students to refrain from violence against others unless physical harm is imminent.

One day Terry was riding the subway in Tokyo. Suddenly a large, belligerent drunk laborer staggered onto the train. He cuffed a woman holding a baby, sending her sprawling. He then tried to kick an elderly woman as she scurried to safety. Terry rose, determined to quickly subdue the drunk. At that moment, a friendly "Hey!" pierced the air. It came from a little old Japanese man sitting next to the drunk and looking at him in a most cordial way. The old man asked the drunk if he had been drinking sake. The drunk bellowed that he had, but it was none of the old man's business. The old man said that he and his wife drank warm sake every night as they sat in the garden and watched the sun set. As the drunk looked into the old man's eyes and tried to follow his conversation about the trees in the garden, his countenance began to soften. The old man asked the drunk if he had a wife with whom to drink sake. The drunken man began to cry as he explained that his wife had died the previous year. It was then that he had taken to drink and had lost his job. Now he was so ashamed of himself. Soon the drunk's head rested in the old man's lap, as the old man stroked his dirty hair. Terry humbly realized that the real master of aikido had resolved the problem with compassion, not muscle.[8]

The attack on the subway arose out of someone's pain. The only remedy for pain is love. Certainly the aikido student would have been justified in taking forceful countermeasures. He might have even done so without hatred. However, the master understood the higher principles of empathy and compassion.

Rather than making contemptuous judgments, consider mitigating circumstances. Like the laborer in the story above, people behaving badly are often expressing pain that they do not know how to handle constructively. Without condoning bad behavior, consider what might have happened in that person's life. The Yugoslavian dictator Slobodan Milosevic lost both parents to suicide as a child. Both Adolph Hitler and Sadam Hussein were exposed to severe brutality as children. Visualize a child who freezes painful emotions and turns to anger to help numb the pain. It is then easier to release hostility. Recall that much anger arises from the deep fear of self-diminishment. Remember that and think, "I wonder if I can help."

6. Look at faces. When someone offends you, focus on the person's face. See a person who is suffering and fallible, just like you. See beneath the distressing disguise of anger and see a person who was once a vulnerable child and is *still* vulnerable. Look for something likeable.

7. Seek evidence of good in yourself. We tend to see others as we view ourselves.

8. Change yourself. We can expect to trust others more easily when we first trust ourselves. A former student with a radiant expression related, "I used to be cynical. I was raised by a distrustful single mom. When I stopped to examine myself and consider I had problems that I'm willing to admit and adjust, I started getting along better with people."

- Replace selfish goals and fears with altruistic ones. Try to help or commit to a good cause. For example, Viktor Frankl volunteered to treat infected concentration camp prisoners rather than meaninglessly vegetate. Join with others in working for a common goal. Do something altruistic. Start small.[9] Help someone, perhaps a stranger, in distress.
- Live up to your moral capacity.

9. Realize that you don't need to maintain a wall of suspicion to protect yourself. When someone offends you, stay calm. See yourself as strong, friendly, and secure (that's the real protection). See

others as well meaning, trying their best according to what they understand to do.

10. View all people alike—as fallible but perfectible and desiring the same thing: to be happy and avoid suffering. Hitler was one who did not grasp this concept. He believed that those who were weak and fallible didn't deserve to live. In his view only superior people deserved to live. Of course he realized in his last year of life that he was fallible, as Germany collapsed under his flawed leadership. He had fits of rage and hid his medical weaknesses. Then he committed suicide. Rather than viewing people with contempt, it is far better to accept people despite their flaws and try to lift them. Two African American students in class told their stories about their most distressing aspect of life, which happened to be discrimination. One, a beautiful, bright-eyed woman, experienced it from other races. The other, a large and gentle man, experienced it from his own race because he was so fair skinned. I asked them how they had avoided bitterness. The first said, "Because we were taught that all people are truly equal." The second said that his father taught him to love everyone. A sense of true equality and acceptance of all humankind is a powerful antidote to hostility.

11. Turn down the hostility dial. Exhibit 11.1 represents a continuum of human emotion.[10] Think how you would feel when the hostility dial is all the way to the right. Now imagine slowly moving the dial to the left. First your respect for others is dutiful and courteous. As the dial moves to the left, your respect becomes more positive in nature. As the dial continues to move left, you begin to feel genuine altruism. Ponder what that would feel like.

12. Be a carrier of kindness. Replace hostile behaviors with respectful ones.[11]

- Compliment rather than criticize. Praise a job well done. Express appreciation.
- Avoid reviling, backbiting, or other disrespectful speaking of others—to their face or behind their back. If it is unkind

Exhibit 11.1 Emotion Continuum

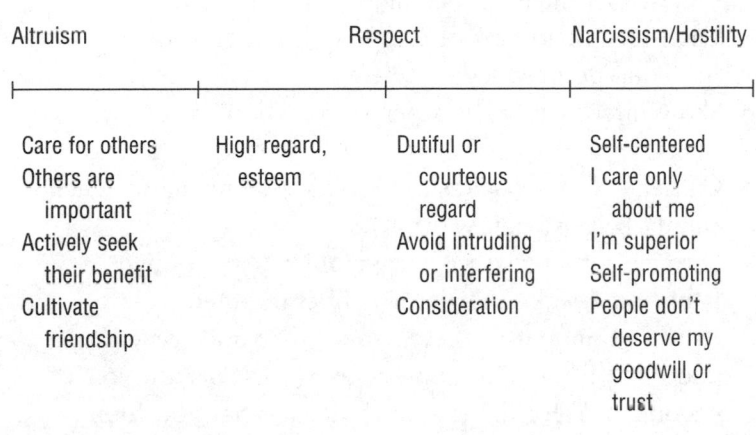

Altruism		Respect	Narcissism/Hostility
Care for others	High regard,	Dutiful or	Self-centered
Others are	esteem	courteous	I care only
important		regard	about me
Actively seek		Avoid intruding	I'm superior
their benefit		or interfering	Self-promoting
Cultivate		Consideration	People don't
friendship			deserve my
			goodwill or
			trust

and unnecessary, don't say it, no matter how justified it seems. Speak respectfully of others and to others. Speak softly and calmly. (This doesn't mean, however, that one can't firmly insist on respectful treatment.)

- Say nice things about people behind their back. Excuse yourself when people gossip or backbite, or be silent.
- Wish others well, even those who offend you. It sometimes helps to realize that they suffer when they are offensive to others. If they knew how to behave better, they probably would.
- Do something without being asked, such as helping with a chore, or giving a hand when someone is frustrated or having a bad day.
- Smile, greet people, ask them about their day. Give a hug. Sit with someone who doesn't have many friends.
- Excuse someone's mistakes.
- Read or work with a child.
- Let someone else have his or her way sometimes.
- Help others get involved or feel included in an activity.

Drills

- View the *Mother Teresa* video, or read a biography of a selfless or principled person.
- Catch people in acts of everyday kindness—or at least behaving politely, legally, etc.
- Show interest in what a person you don't know well is doing.
- Cultivate a new friendship (e.g., ask someone to lunch simply because you want to).
- Consider other reasons to explain a person's bad behavior, besides malice or deliberate intent.
- At the beginning of the day decide to find something good and likeable to appreciate in each person you encounter. Describe in your journal what you found at day's end.
- Actively practice being friendly. Appreciate small reciprocations.
- Look into the eyes of people and smile.[12]

Reflections

Sweetness is not a weakness. Hostility hinders, never helps a career.

(Meyer Friedman)

Ask yourself why you are more likely to notice the weaknesses in others, rather than their good qualities.

(Anonymous)

Do not be too severe upon the errors of the people, but reclaim them by enlightening them.

(Thomas Jefferson)

All friends were once strangers.

(Anonymous)

Judge not, that ye be not judged.

(Matt. 7:1)

We can respond to irritation with a smile instead of a scowl, or by giving warm praise instead of icy indifference. . . . Love, patience, and meekness can be just as contagious as rudeness and crudeness.

(Neal A. Maxwell)

I don't meet all of my own needs. Why should I condemn others for doing the same? In other words, I sure mess up; why should I expect you won't? You're fallible, struggling, suffering, and wanting happiness—just like me.

(Anonymous)

We can also meditate on the suffering of those who cause us to suffer. Anyone who has made us suffer is undoubtedly suffering too.

(Thich Nhat Hanh, *Peace Is Every Step*)

One dies inside when one stops believing in the goodness of mankind. This self-inflicted death can be reversed by taking a fresh look at the evidence and realizing that all humans, though fallible, have some goodness within.

(G. R. Schiraldi)

Love is more powerful, more transforming, than hate.

(Anonymous)

People tend to reflect back the feelings we give them— both good and bad.

(Anonymous)

Love is a fruit in season at all times, and within the reach of every hand.

(Mother Teresa)

No one in his *right* mind joys in another's suffering. So if someone is deliberately offensive, he is ill and deserving of compassion.

(Anonymous)

Look for the helpers. You will always find people who are helping.

> (told to Fred Rogers by his mother, when
> he was frightened by the news)[13]

Suggested Activity

Go through the "Strategies to Reduce Hostility" section. Make a plan to do those things that are most important to you. Then do them.

12

Forgiving

Resentment is like taking poison and waiting for the other person to die.

—Malachy McCourt

DO YOU STILL find yourself reliving past hurts? Do you feel betrayed? Do you dwell on wrongs done to you and not so much on the wrongs you might have done? Do you avoid loved ones? Do you bristle when you hear the names of certain people? Do you blame your dissatisfaction or failures on someone or something—parents or other family members, bosses, or a lover who jilted you? Do you find some pleasure in resentment, perhaps because you feel morally superior to the offender, or perhaps because you justify your present behaviors by things that happened to you in the past? Do you feel cold or unfeeling? Do you find it difficult to trust people? Do you feel you've been victimized?

If the answer to any of these questions is yes, the skill of forgiving might be especially empowering to you. Formerly associated only with spiritual well-being, forgiving has been found to improve physical and mental health as well. Harboring resentment or grudges has been likened to carrying around a cannon on the back, hoping for a chance to retaliate against the offender, who perhaps is not aware of your pain. This wartime mentality fatigues, keeps the focus off life's loveliness, and elevates blood pressure and arousal. As long as people remain on alert, wounds can't heal.

Forgiving might be considered the crown jewel of anger management skills. It is a skill needed for everyday offenses, as well as for unconscionable acts committed by loved ones or people you don't know.

What Is Forgiveness?

Forgiving means that we choose to release resentment, hatred, bitterness, and desires for revenge for wrongs done to us; it is a way to come to peace with the past. In forgiving, we decide to break our troubling connection to the offender. We realize that no offense is worth the price of destroying our peace. Forgiving is taking the arrows out of our gut, rather than twisting them around inside us. We move away from and beyond the offender and the offense and take full responsibility for our present happiness. We choose to forgive so that we will suffer less and be free to live. Sometimes forgiveness might even free the offender to heal and grow. For example, following the Los Angeles riots in 1992, Reginald Denny forgave the rioter who severely and deliberately injured him. He explained that although he was angry, he truly loved the offender. The offender's mother said Denny's response was the first action that softened her son's anger.

Forgiving is a personal choice that does not depend on the offender's deserving it, asking for it, or expressing remorse—although these certainly can make forgiving easier. *Forgiving is about the offended person's inner strength, rather than the offender's. We voluntarily forgive because we realize that getting even does not heal.*

What Blocks Forgiveness?

A number of fears and misconceptions can block us from obtaining the benefits of forgiving.

1. *Forgiving means I am condoning the behavior.* In forgiving we acknowledge and condemn the behavior, but still choose to release hatred and ill will toward the offender. Forgiving is not giving in, giving up power, or lowering your guard. One might choose to work for justice, but without poisoning bitterness.

2. *Forgiving means forgetting.* Forgiving only means that negative feelings are released. Remembering lessons from the past helps us to take prudent precautions in the present. It leads to wisdom, experience, empathy, and compassion.

3. *Forgiving will make the offender think his actions didn't hurt me.* One can clearly make the impact of the behavior known and still release hatred.

4. *Without the anger, I'll be vulnerable.* Without the anger and hatred, you'll be able to identify the hurts and eventually heal them.

5. *Forgiving risks making me look weak.* So what? Inside one knows that forgiving is a sign of strength. No one's negative opinion discounts that. In truth, many will respect one who has the maturity to release the need to retaliate.

6. *If I give up resentment, I'll have to take responsibility for my own happiness. I'll have to change.* True. This is a bit frightening, yet infinitely more rewarding than staying chained to the past.

7. *Forgiving means the loss of purpose.* Sacrificing revenge as a motive frees us to replace it with more constructive purposes.

8. *If I don't make him pay, he'll never change.* When backed into a corner, people usually defend themselves. When confronted with reason (i.e., when people can understand that there is a better way and believe that they can attain it), they are usually more motivated to change. If you determine that justice is required to protect yourself, society, and/or the offender from repeating and reinforcing bad habits, then one can pursue the course of justice with a sense of duty, not hatred.

9. *Forgiving means reconciling or trusting.* Trust requires a belief in the other person's character and must be earned over time in order for a relationship to be rebuilt. It might not be prudent to reconcile or trust in some situations. However, forgiveness can still occur even without reconciling or trusting.

10. *Certain acts are unforgivable.* Since forgiveness is entirely about the internal state of the offended, not the act itself, any act is forgivable. This is where the sense of power derives, from saying, "Even though this was a despicable act, nevertheless I forgive you."

11. *I'll be disloyal to others if I drop the grudge.* There are better ways to show loyalty than by hating.

12. *The offender is all bad and deserving of my animosity.* Offenders are human, weak, in pain, not in their right mind, and/or ignorant. They are already suffering for this, and life will continue to punish them for their imperfections. Maybe you don't need to assume total responsibility for fixing them.

13. *Revenge will restore my peace.* Getting even does not replace what was lost. It only brings the avenger down to the offender's level and makes him or her feel as bad and inhumane.

The Principles of Forgiving

1. *Commit to heal and forgive.* It is said that when one commits, Providence moves.

2. *Expect the act of forgiving serious offenses to be difficult.* It is especially difficult if you don't know how to do it yet. People sometimes think, "Why is this so hard? I should be able to just forgive and release this hurt." That would be nice, but there is nothing easy or natural about forgiving. You're not perfect; you're still learning how to do this. Forgiving serious offenses will likely take time. Per-

haps more healing must occur before forgiveness is completed. Partial forgiveness is showing progress. Some people feel that forgiving certain serious offenses requires divine assistance.

3. *Acknowledge that an offense has taken place and appropriately assign responsibility.* For example, abuse by parents is not the child's fault. Accept that someone who loves you can misbehave. Acknowledge the hurt and the pain. Identify losses so that they may be grieved and wounds might eventually heal. Pennebaker's writing exercise (see page 134) can be an effective medium for this, as is artistic expression or confiding to another trusted person. In constructively identifying and expressing all feelings, the goal is not to rehearse the pain forever but to release the infection and soothe the wound so that it can heal.

4. *If forgiving is difficult, you might try forgiving lesser offenses first.* You might start by making a list of all offenses you have yet to forgive. List them in ascending order, according to the degree of hurt the offense causes. You might start by forgiving lesser offenses before progressing to the deeper ones. Whom might we forgive? A partial list includes:

- Parents for neglect, abuse, failing to protect you, demanding too much, expecting too little, being inconsistent
- Siblings for their all-too-apparent and seemingly inexcusable faults
- Lovers for abandoning or rejecting you
- Teachers for embarrassing you
- Bosses for passing you over or firing you
- Loved ones who died, leaving you feeling abandoned
- People you didn't know who hurt you
- People who discriminated against you based on gender, race, religion, etc.
- Playmates who didn't choose you to be on their team
- Institutions, government, media
- God for allowing bad things to occur

5. *Lower your expectations of the offender*. Someone who was neglectful or abusive previously might not be able or willing to now say the healing words, "I hurt you, I was wrong, I'm sorry." The love needed to facilitate healing might need to come from within and/or from others.

6. *Release the idea that a past offense is responsible for your present unhappiness*. This compounds the pain by keeping one in the helpless victim role. There is a strength in vulnerability, realizing that one can bend but not break; that one can feel pain without turning cold and bitter; that one can commit to restoring happiness after suffering.

7. *Complete emotional business*. In some cases, it is possible to confer with an offender, explaining your feelings and your desire to clear the air. This can be quite healing if the offender is not abusive, ridiculing, or indifferent. But what if the offender has died, is not receptive, is malicious, or denies wrongdoing? A number of strategies, explained in the next section, can still help to complete emotional business.

8. *Forgive yourself* for being vulnerable, for taking offense, for ways you might have contributed to the offense—for being imperfect. You need to give up resentment toward yourself so that you can commit to restoring happiness in your life.

Questions to Help Us Forgive

1. Was the offender intentionally trying to hurt you personally or was his behavior a reflection of his own spiritual illness? Will you make allowances for the offender's upbringing? Do you know what it was?
2. Are you willing to condemn the offender's behavior but not the offender?
3. Are you willing to give up ill will toward the offender and allow others to judge him?
4. Are you willing to shift your focus away from the offense and toward life's loveliness?

5. Are you ready to allow love to heal you? Are you willing to trust again?
6. Are you willing to give up the hurting and hating?

Forgiveness Strategies

The Gestalt Chairs Technique

In order to complete the business of forgiving deeper offenses, your feelings must be acknowledged, expressed, and worked through. Ideally, the offender will listen to and feel the full extent of your pain, acknowledge that wrong was committed, and express sorrow—fully knowing what he/she is sorry about. The offender will not shut you down and minimize your feelings with comments such as, "Oh, I didn't mean it" or "I wasn't trying to hurt you—don't be so sensitive." Gestalt chairs can be used to process unfinished business with an offender who is dangerous, unavailable, or unable or unwilling to deal with your hurt. It can help you to process and complete your feelings, and also, perhaps, better understand the offender's position.

1. Arrange two chairs, facing each other at an angle. Sit in one.
2. Take two easy, deep breaths. Relax. Calm yourself as you prepare to get in touch honestly with your feelings.
3. Imagine the offender sitting in the other chair. Notice what it is like being with this person. Notice your feelings, the anger, and all the other feelings beneath the anger.
4. Begin a dialogue.

   - Start by making a positive statement (e.g., "Years from now I want to have good feelings when I think about you, but right now I don't. My aim is to resolve this, not hurt you.").
   - Explain what you want (e.g., "I want you to hear and understand my hurt and not cut me off with 'I'm sorry' or 'I didn't mean it' before hearing me out.").

- Tell the person what you are thinking and feeling.
  - Describe what happened.
  - Describe the impact of the offense, and especially your feelings (e.g., "I felt . . . ; Now I feel . . .").
- Remain seated. Think. Feel your feelings—the anger, the hurt, the sadness.

5. Change seats. Allow the offender to think and feel his feelings—his own hurts, disappointments, frustrations. Allow the offender to respond. Express the offender's perspective, including his view of what happened, his thoughts and feelings. Stay seated after talking. Think. Feel, as though you were the offender, all his feelings.
6. Keep changing seats until both have fully expressed themselves.

In your mind's eye, look at the person who is listening. Stay with your feelings until they are fully experienced and expressed. At some point, you'll probably want to:[1]

- Check to ensure that what is said was understood. ("Do you understand why this was difficult for me? Are you hearing that?" Then let the other person respond. Both can pose this question.)

- Ask the offender, "I'm trying to understand. What were you feeling? Why did you do that?"

- Consider injecting an opportunity for the offender to say those healing words: "I hurt you. I was wrong. I'm sorry."

- Consider if there were two angry or hurt people, not just one.

You might consider taping such a dialogue to hear the feelings better and further process the dialogue.

Letter of Apology

Some prefer to hear those healing words "I hurt you, I was wrong, I'm sorry" in a letter. You might write yourself an imaginary letter from the offender. In the letter the offender acknowledges the impact of the hurt he caused, explains mitigating circumstances if that will help, and expresses genuine remorse and hopes for your healing and happiness.

Forgiving in Writing

1. Make a list of all the people you have not yet forgiven. For each person, finish these sentences for each offense.

Dear _____,

I felt _____ when _____
　　　　(hurt, angry, etc.)　　　　　　　　　*(describe what happened)*

because _____. I still feel _____.
　　　　　(why you felt as you did)　　　　　　　*(describe present feelings)*

(If possible, add an empathic thought that reflects the other person's state/view at the time, such as: "You were probably feeling pain/insecurity yourself at the time," or "I guess you thought harsh punishment was good discipline." Then, "I want to forgive you.")

Signed, _____

2. After finishing step 1 for each person, complete this statement.

Dear _____,

To the best of my ability, I forgive you for all the hurt you caused me. I release my burden of ill will toward you now, and free you and me to live. (If you shared some responsibility for the offense or carried extreme resentment, you might ask the offender to forgive you, or you might wish to add a statement about forgiving yourself.)

Signed, _____

3. Some people find it useful to ritualistically burn the writings as a symbol of closure.

Forgiveness Imagery

Some people find that imagery is more effective than the rather logical process of writing. Find a comfortable place to relax, take two easy, deep breaths, saying your calming word or phrase on the in-breath and on the out-breath. Then:

1. Identify a loving figure (parent, relative, deity, etc—someone who loves you and makes you feel safe, like a somebody).

2. Think of a person who has offended you. Reflect upon the offense, assigning responsibility for the wrong he/she did.

3. Express your pain in the presence of the loving figure. Physically locate your feelings of rejection, inferiority, violated trust, anger, or other forms of hurt. Give the pain a shape and color. Imagine the love of that loving figure as a bright light, surrounding you and infusing the places that hurt.

4. Imagine the offender's real-life battles (trials, challenges, difficulties). Imagine the adversity he is facing. What is it like to face it? Imagine him as a hurting child, perhaps a victim himself.

5. Imagine his strong points.

6. Can you recall shared good times? Joyful experiences? Ways he supported you or made you feel good? This can sometimes account for part of the difficulty of letting go.

7. Accept responsibility for taking offense.

8. Send your forgiveness and healing to the offender. Imagine something nice happening to him, such as filling the gaps and needs of his childhood. Imagine wishing him well. See him filled with and behaving with loving kindness.

9. Scan your body for remaining hurt or heaviness. Feel it lifting away from your body and taking a shape in front of you. The lov-

ing figure pulls you through the hurt and heaviness, embraces you, and kindly whispers: "The hurting is healing. You are safe, loved, and protected now." You feel your entire body filled with peace.

Drills

- Say "Maybe I'm wrong" several times.
- Try saying, "I was wrong. I'm sorry. Please forgive me."
- Forgive yourself for something you did.
- Practice forgiving people for their trivial mistakes.

Reflections

The more a man knows the more he forgives.

(Confucius)

There is no peace in the nursing of a grudge. There is no happiness in living for the day when you can "get even."

(Gordon B. Hinckley)

If we are willing to look at another person's behavior toward us as a reflection of the state of his relationship with himself rather than as a statement about our value as a person, then we will, over a period of time, cease to react at all.

(Anonymous)

A man that studieth revenge keeps his own wounds green.

(Francis Bacon)

I bear no grudge at all against those who condemned me (to death) and accused me.

(Socrates)

No one in his right mind will knowingly harm another feeling human being.

(Anonymous)

Wisdom always embraces as one of its indispensable components, the processes of pity and forgiveness.

(Anonymous)

One of the most Godlike expressions of the human soul is forgiveness.

(Dallin H. Oaks)

Where is God when it hurts? He is in you, the one hurting, not in it, the thing that hurts.

(Paul Brand, M.D.)

Suggested Activity

Read through the "Forgiveness Strategies" section of this chapter. Complete those strategies you consider important to help you acknowledge your feelings, understand all viewpoints as much as possible, heal, and release the pain.

13

Interpersonal Skills

It isn't that they can't see the solution. It is that they can't see the problem.

—G. K. Chesterton

WITH A VARIETY of anger management skills securely in place, we now turn our attention to skills that build satisfying interpersonal relationships. Most people would say that they desire high-quality relationships with others, yet for many this desire can outweigh their talent, as evidenced by the high rates of divorce and domestic violence.[1] Controlling anger is an important first step. This chapter will explore how these anger regulation skills can be combined with other people skills to result in more satisfying relationships with others, especially family members.

General Rules of Thumb

Whether we are referring to relationships with family members, coworkers, or friends, you'll be more likely to build high-quality relationships if you:

1. *Create an emotional climate that is safe and secure and allows people to be their best.* The attitudes of respect, acceptance, empathy, and compassion prevail. The atmosphere is free of criticism and censure—compliments outweighing criticism by *at least* five to one.

2. *Make understanding others your first priority.* Watch peoples' expressions. Listen to the tone of their voice. Discern if they are receptive to your interest or if they want to be alone. Try to gauge their feelings and understand what is behind them before focusing on being understood.

3. *Actively invest in your social life.* Accept invitations. Plan fun: gatherings, outings, lunch dates, etc. Be interested in people. Ask about their interests.

4. *Remain upbeat.* There is something refreshing about a relationship where honest feelings can be authentically shared, even negative feelings such as sadness, fear, or anger. However, lasting, enjoyable relationships have as their main focus things that are interesting, amusing, and entertaining. Ask yourself, "What am I enthused about?" Then share that.

5. *Show interest in the other person.* This creates bonds and reduces resentment as you share enjoyable times together. Structured meetings can facilitate planning and coordination. One-on-one encounters, such as recreation or informal discussions in the car, are also important.

Couples' Skills

Although most people intend marriage to be a joyous experience, the National Marriage Project reported the percentage of first marriages that were very happy declined from 54 percent in 1976 to 38 percent in 1996. Considerable research[2] indicates that two major factors predict marital satisfaction.

1. *Enjoyment.* Satisfied couples spend time working and playing together, building trust, respect, and joint interests. Their relationship is marked by friendship, unconditional acceptance, laughter, shared control, compliments, commitment, and expressed affection and liking. They tend to use the word "we" when referring to their experiences. They make each other feel important, equal, secure, and not taken for granted. Shared fun permits the couple to be themselves and enjoy relaxed intimacy.

2. *Handling conflict in ways that strengthen the relationship.* Since we don't marry siblings, differences in values—and therefore conflict—is inevitable. This is not all bad, as conflict can lead to growth. It is not the presence of conflict that predicts divorce, but how that conflict is handled. Satisfied couples handle conflict as a team. They engage each other kindly and calmly. They listen to each other and can take criticism without taking offense or becoming defensive. It follows that they avoid provocative gestures, emotions, and words ("You're such an irresponsible slob; why don't you ever help me!"). They are respectful, not contemptuous (e.g., instead of saying, "Why do you waste your time watching football?", they might say, "You enjoy the game while I read or take a nap.")

Satisfied couples tolerate issues that can't be resolved, which occurs in nearly 70 percent of marriages. They seem to understand that it takes at least ten years for high-quality intimacy to develop, which is good because nearly 90 percent of couples who say their marriage is awful will describe it as pretty good or very good five years later. Thus, they tend to hang in during the difficult times and realize that a successful marriage takes effort. I think of one recently married woman who said, "I wish someone had told me how hard it would be, and that there are times when you don't want to be with your spouse." Satisfied couples tend to realize that:

- There will be differences of opinions. My mate won't always like everything I do or all of my attributes.
- There will be times when people who love each other argue, get angry, and even hurt each other's feelings.

- My mate won't satisfy all my needs and isn't responsible for my happiness. I am.
- We won't always feel close.
- We won't always know what is on the other person's mind without asking.
- Steady, comfortable friendship is more predictive of marital success than blissful, intense romance.

Couples Conflict

About what do people argue? Some of the most common issues are money, sex, chores, communication, in-laws, and how time is spent. Deeper issues relate to trust and not feeling respected, loved, or equal.

Researchers at the University of Denver and authors of the acclaimed book *Fighting for Your Marriage*, Markman, Stanley, and Blumberg* described what we call complementary conflict patterns in men and women. In general, men become more aroused by conflict, and find that uncomfortable. So they tend to withdraw from conflict. They prefer that conflict have structure and rules, and be free of emotions.[3] They also tend to want to solve the problem, and use sex as a means to be close to their partner. Women tend to approach problem solving somewhat differently. They tend to consider more feelings and relationship aspects of issues. The process of problem solving is often more important than finding an immediate solution. That is, rather than wanting to be given a solution—which may seem to suggest that they are not capable of solving the problem—they are likely to appreciate a spouse who encourages and supports a richer exploration of the problem. Women tend to want to talk in order to feel close, and avoid physical intimacy until closeness is obtained. Although both genders want the same things (trust, respect, comfortable companionship, inti-

---

*This section, along with the Speaker–Listener technique, the problem-solving model, taking time-outs, and most of the habits of effective couples, is adapted with permission from H. J. Markman, S. M. Stanley, and S. L. Blumberg, "Fighting for Your Marriage," video set, PREP Educational Products, Inc., Denver, CO, 1991. Also adapted from *Fighting for Your Marriage: Positive Steps for Preventing Divorce and Preserving a Lasting Love* (San Francisco: Jossey-Bass, 1994) by same authors. See Appendix B to order these excellent resources.

macy, loyalty, fun, harmony, and teamwork), they typically seek these things somewhat differently. Women tend to consider talking and listening as ways to show caring. Being less verbal, men might prefer holding hands while watching television. What appears to be called for is a method of solving conflict that explores the range of feelings in a calm way before problems are solved—in a way that addresses the needs of both genders. The University of Denver researchers have outlined methods of conflict resolution that are very effective in reducing divorce rates.

*The Speaker–Listener Technique***

So often in the heat of couples conflict the real issue is lost amongst the name-calling, blaming, put-downs, sarcasm, frustration, and anger. The Speaker–Listener technique cools things down so that the real issue can be explored and eventually solved. In fact, the hotter the issue, the more the safety and structure of this technique are needed. The goal of this basic tool is to develop empathy—to see and respect the other person's viewpoint. The rules follow. Remember that the technique is not more important than the spirit the couple brings. Both must be respectful, calm, and positive.

Rules for Both

1. *The Speaker is the focus of attention.* Use any object to designate the speaker (a book, remote control, piece of carpet). If you are not the speaker, you are the listener.

2. *Take turns.* Once the speaker has spoken and is satisfied that he/she is understood—not before—switch roles.

3. *Both parties speak in a quiet, calm, soft tone of voice.*

4. *Don't try to solve the problem.* Instead, have a good discussion where both of you are heard and understood. Focus on dis-

---

** Adapted with permission from Markman et al., 1991, and Markman et al., 1994. See footnote on page 196.

cussing feelings constructively. Problem solving comes later—once a foundation of understanding and teamwork have been established.

Rules for the Speaker

1. *Speak only for yourself.* Express *your* concerns, not your partner's. Describe your viewpoint—how you think and feel about the issue—not how you assume your partner thinks and feels. Mind-reading can intensify the conflict. Use "I" statements ("When you do X in this situation, I feel . . .") or statements such as, "It seems to me that you . . ."

2. *Keep it short/brief.* Keep your statements simple and concise to help your partner understand, and pause to ensure that your partner is understanding you. Don't worry about interruptions, which are against the rules. You'll have the opportunity to say all you need to say.

3. *Give your partner chances to paraphrase.* After talking for a short while, stop and permit your partner to repeat back what you just said. If the paraphrase isn't quite accurate, politely restate your thoughts as you intended them to be heard ("That's not quite what I meant. I meant X. Would you try paraphrasing again, please?"). Persist until you are satisfied the Listener really hears and understands you.

Rules for the Listener

1. *Paraphrase what you hear the speaker saying.* To show that you are listening and understanding, briefly restate what the Speaker said. It's okay to use your own words. ("Sounds like . . . , So you're feeling . . . , What I hear you saying is . . . , Bad day, huh?") Check to see if your paraphrase seems accurate to your partner. If it doesn't (this is normal), permit the Speaker to patiently restate/clarify. Then paraphrase again. You may ask the Speaker, "Would you please repeat/clarify that?" if you don't understand something. Hold off asking other questions until you are the speaker.

2. *Focus on hearing and understanding the Speaker.* If you focus on paraphrasing, you'll listen better. Don't interrupt, disagree, or contradict. Do not indicate displeasure with gestures or making faces. Simply let the Speaker know that you are listening respectfully, understanding, and trying to be a team. You needn't agree with the Speaker. If you disagree, wait until you are the Speaker to tell your side.

*The Problem-Solving Model****

Too often couples attempt to solve problems prematurely. It may not be a solution that is required as much as understanding, validation, or respect. Once both agree that the problem has been fully discussed using the Speaker–Listener technique and both feel fully understood, then time is set aside for conflict resolution.

An agenda is set, where the problem that is being solved is identified. Tackle one issue at a time. People feel competent when they can solve one problem and not be overwhelmed by several all at once. You might identify the problem as a question, such as, "How can we balance my desire to watch football with our need for time together?" The problem-solving model follows these steps:

1. Brainstorm ideas. Identify as many possible solutions as you can. Anything goes. Do not evaluate or rule out any options at this point. This stifles the creativity process. Enjoy yourselves if possible. Try to build on your partner's ideas. One person writes all of the ideas down.

2. Evaluate the advantages and disadvantages of each alternative. Both speak freely here. There is no bargaining or persuading at this point.

3. Agree on the best idea, combination of ideas, or compromise solution.

*** Adapted with permission from Markman et al., 1991, and Markman et al., 1994. See footnote on page 196.

4. Specify details. What will each person do? When will you put the plan into effect? When is a good time to meet again to evaluate how you're doing?

Take Time-Outs****

In athletics, teams take time-outs whenever things are getting out of control. If at any time anger seems to be escalating, it can be very helpful to call a time-out.

1. Explain to your partner, "We need to talk about this, but I'm starting to feel angry. I'd better take a time-out. Let's take a break for _____ (specify an amount of time, usually less than an hour) and then meet again to continue." Some couples use a prearranged signal, with the understanding that all interaction will stop (no last words or following the person who requests the time-out) and that both partners will return in an hour (or some other prearranged time).

2. Use the time-out period to cool down and gain perspective. You can do something active to physically release the arousal, such as clean, take a walk, or shoot baskets. Figure out what's going wrong and what might help.

3. When you return, you might resume talking if both people are ready. Don't force it. You might suggest using the Speaker–Listener technique.

Note: If your partner is getting angry, you might first try saying "I'm willing to talk if we can both use a normal tone of voice. Let's try the Speaker–Listener technique." A time-out can then be taken if that does not work. If you are at work, you might find other ways to cool down, such as a bathroom break to splash your face.

****Adapted with permission from Markman et al., 1991, and Markman et al., 1994. See footnote on page 196.

The Seven Deadly Sins: Enemies of Love

Washington, D.C., psychiatrist and family therapist Dr. E. James Lieberman has identified seven practices that destroy love.[4] Once identified, they can be eliminated.

1. *Violence*. Letting anger all out may work in the psychiatrist's office, but in day-to-day living one must learn to express anger constructively, responsibly, and effectively. Admit hurt feelings; let yourself be vulnerable. Speak calmly without lifting a hand, or leave the room.

2. *Cruelty* is persisting in doing that which disturbs someone else. This includes teasing, being inconsiderate, or failing to correct annoying habits.

3. *Trespassing* is violating or failing to respect another's privacy or individuality. This includes eavesdropping, reading another's mail, forcing sex on an unwilling partner, or insisting on knowing every detail of another's day.

4. *Infidelity* is a violation of trust. This certainly includes sexual infidelity, the breach of an implied promise. Offended spouses feel angry ("I'm replaceable; not important") and, perhaps, pressured to perform better sexually, but anger blocks performance. Infidelity also includes being undependable or inconsistent, including driving too fast, drunkenness (cheapens one's word), lying, breaking promises, smoking in bed, unenforced threats (bluffing), or telling a third person's secrets.

5. *Nagging*, which is asking for the same thing more than twice. Nagging means you are not being heard or respected. When you ask a second time, be sure you are heard and that the request is doable. Maybe compromise or negotiate. If you ask a third time, you risk being ineffective, weak, or hostile. So either quit asking or lower the boom (e.g., go on strike).

6. *Contempt* is expecting too much from your spouse and then looking down your nose when he or she disappoints you. For example, "Where did you get a lamebrained idea like that?" Since we don't always meet our own expectations, how can we deride others for falling short? A climate of respect permits a person to grow more fully than one of contempt.

7. *Indifference* is the opposite of love, not hate. Without responding to another's hurt, anger, or sadness, relationships do not work.

Seven Habits of Highly Effective Couples*****

1. *Structure time for fun and friendship.* It is said that "A friend is glad to see you and doesn't have any immediate plans for your improvement."[5] Plan time to relax and enjoy each other, without trying to fix your partner or give advice. Brainstorm ideas for fun. You might refer to the Pleasant Events Schedule in Chapter 9. Partners might make separate lists of ideas and pick an event from each list on alternate weeks. Plan spontaneity. For example, set aside a day to be together, with only general plans, such as going to the zoo. Let the details evolve as you go.

2. *Keep fun and friendship times off limits from arguments and discussion of issues.* Say, "This is our fun time. How about if we plan to discuss this tomorrow night?"

3. *Have a weekly couples meeting to plan, set goals, anticipate problems, value your partner, and reaffirm commitment to each other.* One extremely diligent officer at the Pentagon found it very aggravating to return from work and be confronted with a list of demands from his wife. I asked, "Have you ever considered a couples meeting at the beginning of the week—you know, to anticipate

***** Adapted with permission from Markman et al., 1991, and Markman et al., 1994. See footnote on page 196.

problems?" He said, "That's a really good idea. I never thought of that." He also learned to ask for a few minutes of time to unwind when he first got home. Then he could more calmly discuss any problems that had come up that day.

4. *Use the problem-solving model.* Remember to first make sure the problem is fully discussed and understood before trying to solve it. As you're trying to resolve conflict:

- Think of the problem as an "it," a situation to resolve, rather than as a personal attack.
- Try to view your spouse, as respected psychiatrist Aaron Beck has advised, as "vulnerable and upset, not hostile and menacing."[6]
- State your requests in specific—not vague—positive terms (e.g., "Dear, I'd like to spend more time with you on the weekends," rather than "Why don't you show you care?").

5. *Praise and appreciate your partner at every opportunity for:*

- Trying things out
- Listening
- Attempting to improve the marriage
- Being committed

Try saying words such as: "Thanks." "Nice job." "I really like the way you do that." "I really appreciate the way you . . ."

6. *Practice forgiving and seeking forgiveness.* Try to see your partner's point of view. If one sincerely apologizes and understands your hurt, freely forgive. Try to focus on what the partner is doing constructively, rather than the ways he or she is falling short.

7. *Seek to earn cooperation and respect, rather than demanding or trying to control.*

- Honor your spouse's input.
- Create an atmosphere where your partner can flourish for his or her benefit, not yours.

- Be sure your partner knows that he or she is the most important person in your life.
- Ask, "What can I do to help?" (A home is a shared responsibility. Think beyond traditional roles.)
- Sacrifice some personal pleasure in order to help or spend time with your spouse.
- Show extra love after you have a conflict, so that your spouse knows that your bond is secure.
- Don't belittle or use sarcasm that is really thinly veiled criticism.
- Remember that "cool and masterful" is more likely to prevail than violence or arousal.

Family Skills and Practices

The rules for satisfying relationships within the family basically parallel the rules for satisfying couples relationships. Children tend to emulate the practices they see in their parents. If they see their parents respecting each other, they will learn to respect each other. For example, Ron, a successful man who had traveled the world in his work and raised five secure and happy children, related: "Growing up, we were taught never to hit siblings or a spouse. In fifty-one years of marriage, I never saw Dad raise a hand or his voice. I did see hugs, kisses, and Mom and Dad dancing around the kitchen." The following principles and skills can be extended to the family.

1. *Cultivate the family-as-team ethic.* Remind children, "We have to work as a team—we need to work together." Many assume that the purpose of chores is to complete the work. A larger purpose is to build relationships. Lucky children will grow up working alongside their parents.

2. *Hold weekly family meetings or home evenings.* Like couples meetings, these meetings can be used to inform, plan, solve prob-

lems, teach, play or work together, and encourage. One couple created the tradition of using one meeting a month to share goals that each individual had set. Each person went in turn and said something like, "I set out to do X and I was 25 percent successful." Then everyone cheered. There was no criticism or censure, only delight in the progress. Calendars were also coordinated so that no one was surprised during the week.

You might try posting an agenda. Family members can add problems they would like the family to solve, as long as they provide tentative solutions. This teaches the good business skill of suggesting solutions, not just complaining about problems. Then the entire family can brainstorm. All ideas are accepted as having merit with a positive spirit and good humor. You never know what will emerge as the best solution.

Try to balance problem-solving meetings with fun evenings. Just as with couples, families need fun and friendship time where enjoyment, not problems, is the focus.

3. *Plan regular one-on-one parent/child interviews.* Such interviews tend to promote a positive atmosphere and ward off problems. Droubay has described this process.[7] The basic rule of thumb is that the child gets to talk about anything, free of censure and criticism. The parent asks, "What do you need to talk about?" Once children learn they can speak freely, they'll continue to share thoughts and more serious concerns as they grow older. Droubay reports that his three-year-old child was uncertain at first. So he told him, "All I want to do is give you a kiss and a hug and tell you how much I love you." He came running and thereafter insisted on his regular weekly interview. Trying to reinforce patient behavior in another child, he asked, "How come you're so sweet lately?" The child replied, "'Cause I'm so important in our family," and then gave him an unexpected hug. Following a discussion of a challenging problem, his nine-year-old daughter told her mother, "You ought to go in there. Daddy is really a good problem solver." Aside from asking an occasional question, Droubay had only listened to his child talk.

4. *Correct children in private as much as possible.* Try to do so firmly and quickly, then be sure the child knows he or she is accepted so that resentment does not build.

5. *Constructively assert expectations and preferences.* The formula is (a) make a positive statement; (b) describe your feelings related to another's behaviors; then (c) state your preferences. For example, recall the officer who could command his troops but not his boy. He learned to assert without anger: "I really love you and I don't want to be nagging you. But I get upset when you return the truck without cleaning it. I'd like you to pick up the trash inside and hose it down after your date. Will you do that?" His son responded, "Sure, Dad. I didn't realize that mattered so much to you." Had his son not honored his request, he could have stated the consequences (and followed through): "If you don't clean the truck after you use it, I won't permit you to use it for a month."

6. *Teach children to solve their own problems.* Rather than trying to solve siblings' problems for them, try viewing their repeating conflicts as opportunities for them to learn conflict resolution skills. Put the responsibility on their shoulders. Let them know that you know they are capable of solving their own problems. For example, consider the following situation. Two teenage siblings were constantly bickering over who got to choose which television shows to watch. Eastman suggests the following guidelines:[8]

- Avoid futile questions (e.g., "Why can't you get along?" "Whose turn is it?" "Who started this commotion?").
- If the situation is out of control (in this case the siblings were actually screaming at each other and getting into physical fights), then considerable structure is probably necessary. The parents might call a family meeting and explain: "We think that you are old enough to settle your differences. We expect you to do so civilly. If you successfully resolve the problem, you will continue to enjoy the privileges of living here, including the privilege

of watching television. If you choose to scream, hit, or
retaliate in a destructive way, you will deny yourselves the
following privilege . . . "[9]

- The steps of problem solving are explained: select one problem, brainstorm solutions, evaluate each solution, select the
best solution, and specify the details. Parents might explain
the use of a problem-solving planning sheet (see Exhibit
13.1). On this sheet, the problem is clearly stated, along
with the objective (e.g., to equally and respectfully share
television privileges). Possible solutions are listed, then the
advantages and disadvantages of each one. The solution that
seems best to both siblings is specified, along with the details
of who is to do what and when. (If no solution were mutu-
ally agreeable, then more brainstorming would be required.)
In addition to reinforcing good behavior with praise (e.g., a
simple, "It's great to see you getting along nicely"), parents
may provide additional incentives for desirable behavior
(e.g., "If harmony is maintained for a week, then . . . [movie
tickets, no dishes on Friday night, restoration of previously
revoked privileges, etc.].").[10] The consequences are also specified for one party's violation of the plan (e.g., doing the
other sibling's chores for the day). Both siblings sign and
date the form. A review date is also specified, which permits
the siblings to evaluate how well the plan is working and to
make needed adjustments. Treat the agreement like a contract and post it where all the family can see it.

Here's the way the problem-solving process unfolded. The siblings each made a list of their favorite shows and times. For times
when there was disagreement, they brainstormed that they could
alternate who gets to choose (1) by nights or (2) by weeks. As they
problem solved, the idea emerged that the sibling who wasn't watching his favorite show could go to the mall with friends, learn a
hobby, read, etc. They also came up with a barter system, whereby
one sibling could watch an additional show on an off night in
exchange for doing a chore, provided the other sibling agreed.

Exhibit 13.1 Problem-Solving Planning Sheet

Problem: _____

Objective: _____

Possible Solutions:

Plan A _____
                         Pros   Cons

Plan B _____
                         Pros   Cons

Plan C _____
                         Pros   Cons

The Solution That We Think Is Best (circle the plan above or write a modified plan here):

_____

_____

Specifics: Who Does What, When, How Long

_____

_____

Rewards: _____

Consequences: _____

Review Date: _____

Signed: _____ Date: _____

          _____ Date: _____

Drills

- Ask about another's activities for the day and listen quietly.
- Express affection verbally.
- Compliment a loved one or a coworker.
- Ask, "Is there anything I can do for you?"
- Do something nice for a member of your family.
- Frequently say, "That's a good point," or "I never thought of that."
- Next time you are tempted to complain or criticize a loved one, fill the person with love. Fill yourself with love. Say, "I understand. Thanks for all you do. I love you."

Reflections

There should be no yelling in the home unless there is a fire.

(David O. McKay)

The most important work (you'll ever do) is within the walls of your own home.

(Harold B. Lee)

Happiness in the home will lead to happiness in the world.

(Dalai Lama)

Take away love and our earth is a tomb.

(Robert Browning)

Only a life lived for others is worth living.

(Albert Einstein)

Govern a family as you would cook a fish—very gently.

(Chinese proverb)

Your money doesn't kiss you back.

(Anonymous)

Suggested Activities

1. Apply the Speaker–Listener technique to a somewhat difficult issue until both partners are satisfied that the issue is understood. Then apply the problem-solving method, taking time-outs as needed.
2. Schedule spontaneous fun time with a loved one.
3. Schedule and then hold weekly couples meetings, family meetings, and parent/child interviews.

14

Innovative Approaches

You don't want to stand rigid like a tall oak that cracks and collapses in the storm. Instead, you want to be flexible, like a reed that bends with the storm and survives.

—Deepak Chopra

IN THIS CHAPTER we'll explore two techniques that will allow you to quickly and effectively apply the skills you've learned so far: HEALS and the ASSIST Program. Then we'll explore humor, which helps us view hooks from a lighter perspective, and affirmations, which reinforce the mind-set of calmness.

HEALS

Developed by psychologist Steven Stosny,[1] the HEALS method affords a rather easy-to-remember way to manage anger under pressure. Initially, try this with a hook that is manageable; for example, your partner watches TV when you have a problem and want to talk. Notice the signs that tell you that you are angry, such as tight shoulders or stomach, clenched fists, or raised voice. Then follow these five steps, which create the acronym HEALS:

1. **Healing.** See the word *Healing* flash three times in bright colors in your mind.

2. **Experience** the deepest hurt.

- Say slowly, "I feel . . . (insignificant, unimportant, rejected, disregarded, devalued, mistrusted, powerless, unlovable, etc.)." The last may be the deepest and most difficult feeling to acknowledge.
- Feel the feeling for a second or two. Without feeling, there is no healing.
- Think of yourself as so vast that you can let hurts in.

3. **Apply compassion** to heal the hurt.

- Remind yourself that it is natural to feel upset, hurt, frustrated, etc.
- Think about an image that connects you to your core value. Try to identify an image that counters each deepest hurt. For instance, if you feel unlovable, identify a time when you felt loved or accepted, were treated with kindness, etc. If you feel powerless, identify a time when you felt capable, constructively powerful, etc. Examples of such images include:

  - A compliment or expressed appreciation from a loved one.
  - Being embraced by a child, a loved one, or God.
  - Simply being with a trusted friend.
  - Being in a sacred place and feeling "at home" or safe and protected.
  - A time when you felt competent, brave, accomplished, kind, creative, in control, etc.
  - You might also refer to the core worth meditation in Chapter 7.[2]

- The image may be strengthened with an appropriate statement, such as "I am worthwhile" or "I am powerful/capable/lovable" or "God really will take care of me."

4. **Love yourself** by feeling compassion for the offender.

- Identify the core hurt of the offender. Ask, "Why would someone behave that way?" Often the offender is feeling the same hurt that you are feeling under your anger.
- Try to feel the good feeling of meeting his anger with your compassion. Think about his core value and the things you share as human beings (the same fears, hurts, needs). When you do so, you'll feel more connected to others and yourself, and more powerful and in control.

5. **Solve** the problem by taking action when you can. This might mean:

- Setting up a couple's meeting or family council to problem solve.
- Setting limits or disciplining your child.
- Forgiving—releasing bitterness, whether or not the offender asks for it or deserves it—so that you can be freed from your suffering.
- Seeking help if you lack the skills to solve the problem.
- Asserting (e.g., "I don't let anyone treat me disrespectfully, not even you."). Then leave the person alone to mull things over. Remember, do your best, speak from the heart, and don't get too attached to the outcome.
- Distract. After processing and learning from it, try to forget about it (i.e., think about other things, so as not to stew).

At first, try using HEALS in quiet times, such as during a time-out period or at the end of the day. Do it repeatedly until you can do it automatically under pressure. Stosny recommends practicing HEALS twelve times per day for six weeks.

State of Washington ASSIST Program

We have the greatest respect for those who can make complex skills so simple that even children can understand and apply them. To do so means that the teacher really understands the principles. Pat Huggins, clinical instructor in counseling at the University of Washington, has developed an effective and simple anger management program for children that is widely used throughout the Northwest. These simple skills, we have found, are also effective for adults. The ASSIST Program[3] rests on the principle that "It's okay to be mad. It's not okay to be mean." A basic tool in the program is the turtle trick. When the turtle is threatened, it goes into its shell, where it is warm and safe. We can pretend that we can pull into a safe shell to calm down and think for a little while—take some easy, deep breaths, relax, and think.

The Four Steps

1. *Stop and calm down.*

- Pay attention. At the first cues of anger, simply tell yourself, "Stop."
- Do the turtle trick. Go into the warm, safe shell. Relax, take some deep breaths, and think:
  - Is it worth getting mad?
  - It's not such a big deal.
  - I can control my anger.
  - Stay calm. Don't let this get you in trouble.
  - It won't pay to lose my temper.
  - Figure out a plan before you do anything rash.
  - I can't expect other people to be the way I want.[4]

2. *Think about the best thing to do.* Start by asking, "How much anger can I show without causing myself trouble?" Then ask, "What's the best thing to do here?" The options are:

- Stay and either ignore the problem (Ask: Was it deliberate? Is this a big deal? Will this matter in a few days?) or deal with the problem/person.
- Walk away. Simply leave or take a time-out.
- Seek help.

3. *Talk it over*. Trying to hide the anger and keep it in makes us seem different, less fun, keeps people away. Putting it into words so we don't explode saves embarrassment, hurt, etc. Your choices are:

- Talk directly with the person; explain why you're angry (so they know what you feel) and what you want (e.g., to change the situation, prevent it from recurring, improve the relationship). Some options are:

  - I'm really upset. I'll talk to you later about this.
  - I don't like it when you . . . . I'd feel better if you didn't do that.
  - That's bothering me. Would you stop?
  - Cut it out.
  - I'd like you to do X. You're doing Y. Please do X.
  - I really like it when you do X, but I am bothered by . . .
  - I know you're just teasing, but . . .

- Talk with someone you trust to gain insight and release tension. This is wise if your anger is too strong or the person you are mad at is not receptive. Tell yourself, "I'm going to seek out someone to talk to. In the meantime I won't let it bother me."

- Talk it over with yourself. When things calm down, or in a time-out, try expressing your thoughts and feelings in a journal or through an artistic medium, such as clay. Think about what you feel and want. You might wish to write a card or letter.

4. *Feel good again*. The purpose of this step is to release lingering tension and get beyond the anger.

- Pat yourself on the back. Examples:

  - That was challenging, but I did it.
  - All in all, not bad.
  - I coped with that pretty well.

- That was a difficult situation, hard for a lot of people.
  You did your best, now forget it.
- A mistake doesn't mean I'm without hope.

- Try nonaggressive physical activities—such as exercise
  (biking, running, swimming), cleaning, gardening, folding
  laundry—and other pleasant activities—such as art or
  other hobbies, cooking, reading, listening to music, going
  to a quiet place, pleasant imagery, relaxation exercises, or
  self-talk ("I'm not perfect, but I'm trying.").
- Try to forgive; try to understand the person. You might
  think:

  - Maybe he was mad at the world today, not me.
  - Maybe she didn't know a better way to handle her hurt
    or anger.
  - I don't expect people to be perfect all the time.
  - I forgive you, but I'm really mad—I don't want you
    messing around with my things.

- Forgive yourself. Without making excuses, understand
  your limits (difficult situation, inexperience, ignorance,
  pain, fatigue, etc.). Think:

  - I know I'm not perfect.
  - Everyone makes mistakes.
  - Put it behind me.
  - Plan to make better decisions in the future.

- Tell the person you're mad at:

  - What you did hasn't happened often.
  - I know you are usually thoughtful.
  - We all make mistakes. Let's forget it.
  - I know it's hard.
  - I appreciate your listening and trying.

To gain mastery, one can practice this four-step approach in a
group of three people. One is the angry person, one is the offender,
and the third is a coach. Roles can be rotated.

Humor

Humor is a potent addition to your anger management toolbox. A Jewish tradition states that God called Adam and Eve back before they left the Garden of Eden and gave them a sense of humor to help them get through life with composure—grace under pressure. I've been impressed that each resilient WWII survivor I've interviewed, without exception, deemed humor an essential survival skill. A sense of humor and the ability to laugh together is often cited as an important ingredient of happy marriages.

Humor breaks the spell of overseriousness, that hallmark of mental illness. Being able to laugh at the ridiculous things we do sometimes is an important step in healing. Humor changes our perspective on life. It breaks the grip of fear and pain, expanding our outlook to optimism, acceptance, fun, and play. It is difficult to feel powerless when we feel alert and amused; thus humor also confers a sense of mastery.

Humor is also a social lubricant. It helps us connect to others and provides a service when we help others see the lighter side. Of course, laughter confers numerous health benefits. Laughter provides a physical release that reduces stress hormones. Thus reductions in blood pressure and improvements in immune functioning are some of the health benefits of humor. Let's explore some specific applications of humor as it relates to anger management.

Deflecting the Absurd

Sometimes people, for their own nutty reasons, make absurd statements that don't really call for a serious, reasoned response. An equally absurd deflection might more effectively defuse the situation. The humorous responses shown in Table 14.1 are adapted from the creative work of Mitchell H. Messer, founder of Chicago's The Anger Institute.[5]

Seeing the Lighter Side

When provoked, we could choose to think, "That dirty so and so!" Or we might think: "That poor person needs a nap. Or a mommy.

Table 14.1 Diffusion Techniques

Absurd comment	You reply . . .	And you think to yourself . . .
You're stupid.	There's a lot of that going around. Thanks for drawing that to my attention. I don't know how you stand it.	I won't take your put-down too seriously. I'm not perfect, but I am certainly reasonably smart. I've gotten this far, haven't I? Anyway, you're not qualified to diagnose.
Why are you so stupid?	I was absent that day. Why do you ask?	Even though I'm not a rocket scientist, I'm still a worthwhile person who has a right to learn.
You're just like your mother!	Whose mother should I be like?	I'm really not my mother. I'm separate. I'm trying my best to move beyond her imperfect example.
I don't understand you.	You're right. You don't.	It's not my problem that you don't, and it's not my responsibility to help you see the light. It's certainly okay that we see things differently.
I'm only teasing/berating you because I love you.	You mean the more you love someone, the more you can beat up on them? I didn't realize that love excuses lack of tact.	Love doesn't entitle someone to hurt another and is not an excuse for lack of discretion.
Why are you so inept?	How in the world did you know that? Do you hate it? Doesn't it just *kill* you?[6]	We both know that I won't let your put-downs succeed. Come on, being fallible isn't the end of the world.
You're putting on some pounds.	Speaking of attractive people . . .	I can deflect by changing the subject. I don't need to be needled.
All you have to do to get married is . . .	It's so simple. Why didn't I think of that?	I'm glad you've figured it out for yourself. This is difficult, and I'm still working on it.

Maybe he's constipated, or maybe the poor fellow has a brain tumor." In fact, we might have no idea why our fellow traveler is suffering or behaving badly at the moment, but humor helps us shift the hot thoughts to gentle clarity and acceptance.

Humorously exaggerating the situation can help us uncover the distortions. Try this approach, suggested by Kassinove,[7] the next time you are prone to negatively label someone. If you think someone is a butthead, try to imagine what a butthead would look like. You might try to draw one, a poor person whose brain is replaced by another anatomical part. This also works with dirtball, bonehead, and other varieties of labels. Or consider the organized conspiracies that are perpetrated to intentionally goad us. Have you ever noticed that you always get in the slow line? That's because employees are positioned to be on the lookout for you. When they see you coming, they tell all the checkout personnel, "Quick, whatever line this person gets in, make sure you go extremely slowly." A similar phenomenon occurs when you get in the slow lane of traffic.

You can also exaggerate the catastrophizing distortion. The next time you are in a disagreeable situation, try saying aloud, "Oh, no! This is awful. I just can't stand it. I'm going to hold my breath and have a nervous breakdown right this minute. I *need* a certificate guaranteeing me perpetual serenity." Does it feel horrible to feel insecure? It's not so bad, really. Try the Insecurity Jig. Next time you feel insecure, stand up, throw you hands up in the air, wiggle your fingers, and jump up and down, shouting gleefully, "I'm insecure!" See if your laughter doesn't dispel the pain somewhat.

Exaggerating puts the lie to many distortions. For example, "Thanks for the invitation, but I never go to Orioles games because they always lose when I watch" (personalizing). "Why are you so happy when your life is as bad as mine?" (Irritation fixation.) Rosenblatt humorously helps us counter mind reading and personalizing in his Rules for Aging.

Yes, I know, you are certain that your friends are becoming your enemies; that your grocer, garbage man, clergyman, sister-in-law, and your dog are all of the opinion that you have put on weight, that you have lost your touch, that you have lost your mind; furthermore, you are convinced that everyone spends two-thirds of every day commenting on your disintegration, denigrating your work, plotting your assassination. I promise you: Nobody is thinking about you. They are thinking about themselves—just like you.[8]

There is often some truth in humor. We recall a cartoon wherein a newscaster in effect stated, "In world news tonight, a few bad apples caused all the others to squirm." This cartoon makes one think. It really is the minority of people that behave poorly most of the time, and it is perhaps simplistic to assume that a person is either all good or all bad.

Humor as a Social Lubricant

The story is told that Edwin Stanton had publicly called Abraham Lincoln "a low cunning clown . . . the original gorilla." Lincoln appointed him to be Secretary of War anyway because he felt Stanton was the most qualified person. When friends reported that Stanton had called Lincoln a fool, even after Stanton was a cabinet member, Lincoln responded, "Did he call me that? Well, I reckon it must be true then, for Stanton is generally right." To chuckle at our own imperfections is not only an act of courage, it is an act of wisdom. It stops the tit-for-tat spiral of hatred and models what hostile people often find difficult to internalize: acceptance. Such a response can sometimes defuse hatred and win people over. In fact, at Lincoln's funeral, Stanton sobbed, "There lies the greatest ruler of men the world has ever seen."[9]

Agreeing with our critics can defuse the criticism. In response to "You're putting on weight," you might respond, "Yes, I'm horizontally challenged." To "You're too serious," you might agree and exaggerate, "I resemble that remark. In fact, I'm so serious I'm hiring Jerry Seinfeld as a consultant."[10]

Roberto was a short, slight man from Guatemala who was well liked by his factory coworkers because they knew he cared for them. One day as he pulled in to the factory parking lot he saw two men squaring off. He knew that one carried a gun and feared for the safety of his friends. He related, "I stepped between them, grabbed them by their shirts, and shouted, 'Look, if you two don't cut it out I'm going to take my belt off.'" The two men, either of whom could have crushed Roberto, looked at him, then looked at each other and smiled at the absurdity of the situation. Humor had defused the situation in large part because they knew Roberto cared.

Humor can sometimes soften difficult people. When I would get ornery at West Point (which, of course, was very rare), my kind and dear roommate Tim Rucker would say with feigned pity, "You can't help it." I would laugh at my silliness, knowing that beneath Ruck's humor was a sense of decency and respect for all people, including me. Steve Allen used to say to people who disagreed with him, "Well, you're certainly entitled to your ridiculous opinion." This worked because people knew that Steve liked them.

Of course, relating funny stories about yourself or the general foibles of human nature tends to bond people. The listener thinks, "She's just like me; she understands." It can also be helpful to get an angry person to laugh, if possible, or to change the subject.

The Rules of Humor

Humor may be a partially inborn gift, but it is also a skill that can be cultivated. The rules are simple:

1. *Try to be kind*. Commiserate, don't humiliate. Ensure that the person is enjoying your attempts at humor. (Simply ask, "I was just trying to use some humor. Was that okay?") If you are teasing, be sure that the other person feels accepted and well regarded. Like sex, the best humor is preceded by love. Good humor is good-natured and infused with dignity and acceptance. Sarcasm generally incites resentment and a desire to seek revenge. It is therefore rarely useful.

2. *Don't overuse humor*. Be flexible. Sometimes there is a need to seriously confront other people or our own pain. Don't mask pain and don't use humor as an excuse for not confronting others when necessary.

3. *Find your own style.* Some people are spontaneous and outgoing. Others are low key, watchful, and bemused. Some tell jokes or make others laugh in other ways; others simply appreciate the absurd and laugh at it.

Affirmations

Some people enjoy the way that affirmations reinforce learning. The theory is that mentally rehearsing principles strengthens the neural pathways associated with them, more deeply implanting the ideas and making them available for coping under pressure. The procedure is straightforward. Find a place to relax undisturbed for about fifteen minutes. Deeply relax your body. Take two easy, deep breaths, saying your calming word or phrase to yourself as you breath in and out. Simply read the first statement and allow it to sink in. You might think of a time when you actually believed that statement and acted on it. Or you might imagine what your life would be like if that statement were part of your thinking. Imagine how you would feel and behave. Repeat the statement again; let it roll around in your mind. Feel free to modify or add to the following list of affirmations:

1. I gain advantage by remaining calm and cool under difficult circumstances.
2. I keep a cool, level head when situations get tough and think of the best thing to do.
3. If I find myself feeling angry, I think, "That's okay, that's life," and quickly regain my composure.
4. Although people have hurt me in the past, these hurts do not affect the way I live my life today.
5. I respect all people.
6. I wish kindness and the best interest of all people, including those who have hurt me.
7. I carefully preserve my peace.
8. I let go of bitterness so I can enjoy my life.
9. When I feel my sense of power slipping away, I think, "I still have much power within me to do good."

10. I accept that things don't always go the way I'd like—that I don't always get my way.
11. I accept others, even when they disappoint me.
12. I can laugh at the ridiculous things I do sometimes.
13. I can laugh at the ridiculous things others sometimes do.
14. I have compassion for people, but not necessarily their behavior.
15. I see beyond irritating situations. I know they won't last forever.
16. I try my best, and I don't get too attached to the outcome.
17. I channel anger into constructive actions.
18. When others threaten or intimidate me, I stay calm and secure like a majestic mountain in a storm.
19. Even though others may not like me or treat me well, I love and accept myself.
20. Your own affirmations:

_____

_____

Drills

- Laugh at something you do that is ridiculous.
- The next time someone behaves badly, think or say, "That poor person needs a nap."

Reflections

A friend must not be injured, even in jest.

(Syrus)

It's okay to be mad. It's not okay to be mean.

(Pat Huggins)

If you can laugh at it, you can survive it.

(Bill Cosby)

Suggested Activities

1. Practice HEALS and/or ASSIST repeatedly until they becomes automatic. Record your experience in your journal to solidify your skills.
2. In order to reinforce your learning, practice the affirmations daily for a week or longer.

15

Special Situations: Road Rage, Criticism, and Other Vexations

If you are patient in one moment of anger, you will escape a hundred days of sorrow.

—Chinese proverb

IN THIS CHAPTER we'll explore four situations that can especially challenge your anger management skills: road rage, criticism, discrimination, and frustrations related to loss of control.

Road Rage

Do you remember how thrilling it was to take a spin in an automobile when you were a child? Do you remember how much fun learning to drive was? Is driving still a source of pleasure or has it become an irritating chore?

What's Happened?

Violent driving incidents have increased dramatically in recent years. In such incidents angry drivers try to kill or injure other drivers following a traffic dispute, using everything from guns and knives to fists, canes, and even their own vehicles as weapons. Nearly half of all such incidents are perpetrated by women.

Over half of all highway deaths are at least partially due to road rage. Road rage is excessive anger over traffic conditions. It can range from ruining one's own peace or the peace of the passengers to risky or hostile, aggressive acts against other drivers. What's going on? Why have modern roads become so dangerous?

- Today's roads are more congested. While the number of roads has remained about the same in recent years, the number of cars and the miles driven per driver have increased. This increases the exposure of the average driver to risky, aggressive, or discourteous driving. In congested areas, in fact, the average driver will likely encounter at least one such event per week. In congested traffic, the body remains still for longer periods, unable to expend the energy of fight or flight. So stress and anger can build.

- There are more illegal weapons carried by today's drivers.

- Our sedentary society, with its reliance on services and technology, leaves more and more individuals feeling powerless and not in control. A car can afford a feeling of power and invincibility—and a feeling of rage when one's ability to drive undisturbed is blocked. A car also isolates one from others. A feeling of anonymity counters the feeling of community that sometimes holds aggression in check. It's easier to be cruel to a stranger than a person you know. The invincible driver might feel like a vigilante, able to enforce presumed infractions in ways that would normally be unthinkable outside of the car's protection.

- Advertisements help to create an expectation of unchecked speed. Think of an ad showing a car racing around a mountain road.

- In a culture of cruelty, drivers are more likely to lose their manners and their tempers.

- Our high-stress society tends to create the perception that there is too much to do in too little time. People expect to do more and plan less time for delays. When people drive hurriedly, judgment is likely to be impaired.

What Triggers Road Rage?

Traffic congestion might start the blood boiling. The temperature can then be turned up by other drivers who:

- Speed
- Drive too slow
- Fail to move out of the passing lane
- Weave in and out, crossing lanes
- Cut in front of you
- Take your parking space
- Take out their anger on you
- Make hostile gestures or glare at you
- Yell or curse at you
- Sit on the horn
- Brake quickly or stomp on their brakes to annoy
- Flash their high beams from behind
- Brandish a weapon
- Pass you on the shoulder
- Run red or yellow lights or stop signs
- Rubberneck
- Race or compete
- Make illegal turns
- Close the gap, preventing you from entering the lane

Notice that many of these traffic hooks can threaten the safety of yourself, your family, or others. Many of these hooks lead one to feel diminished (disrespected, disregarded, powerless, etc.). Some only jeopardize one's expectations (e.g., arriving on time or traveling without disruptions). Notice that when *we* do these things, others might react angrily.

One might react by pounding on the steering wheel. Or one might retaliate with hostile or reckless acts, as the incident escalates. Soon the offended is locked in a battle with the offender, which frequently ends in injury or death.

Road rage in a sense is a microcosm of modern living. While the hooks and conditions might be slightly different, the basic issues are still the same. People behave badly. People feel frustrated, threatened, and diminished. People try to feel powerful with anger. However, road rage is no more effective in the long run than any other form of problem anger. And it might be more dangerous.

How Is Road Rage Reduced?

The roadway is a great place to practice your anger skills. Given the confluence of stressful conditions, it might be considered an acid test of anger management skills.

• Beautify your driving environment and enjoy the trip (like children do). Clean the car and make sure the air conditioner is functioning. Turn off the cell phone, as well as loud, pounding music, which can be arousing. Instead listen to soothing music or favorite comedy routines. Beautify your inner environment, as well. Take some easy, deep breaths before starting out, reminding yourself to be compassionate and patient. Rather than waiting to relax after you arrive, relax as you travel. Don't poison your environment with hatred, competition, or a dangerous race to save time. Make the journey itself enjoyable. Determine to be a source of pleasure to those around you, rather than a source of frightening anger. Enjoying life and time with your loved ones is more important than punishing another driver or saving a few minutes.

• Drive at a leisurely rate. Ask, "Will the ten minutes I save by driving like a madman really matter?"

• Leave early, allowing extra time for delays. Challenge the belief that arriving early will be unpleasant. Plan something to enjoy when you arrive early—visiting with people, studying faces/a playbill/clouds, having a conversation, or simply being with a loved one.

• Be actively kind, courteous, and polite. Try to look at the faces of other drivers with respect. View them as fallible, suffering people, just like yourself.

• Let the police take care of policing (i.e., enforcing the law). Maybe I don't have to punish or teach a lesson. Making others pay only escalates anger since they don't accept me as an authorized police officer or teacher. They're unlikely to appreciate my "lesson" since I'm not the highway sheriff.

• Be flexible. Be like a tai chi master who wins by yielding and bending to the power of others in a controlled, powerful way. Know that you can use your power in more constructive ways. Yield to others. Intentionally let someone in front of you. Courtesy is not a weakness.

• Don't swallow the hook. Refuse to react to aggressive or risky driving.

• Keep your identity separate from your car. Remember that when you step out of the car, you'll still be fallible, human, and worthwhile. Your worth does not equal your car. Don't let the car change your identity. Don't do anything in your car that you wouldn't do face to face with someone who is bigger or better armed (he or she may well be).

• Think in new ways, rather than locking into old thought patterns. If someone is driving badly, ask why he would be doing that. Maybe he's not doing it intentionally. Maybe he's lost, old, inattentive, preoccupied, confused, troubled, in pain, running late, rushing to the hospital, not playing with a full deck, or unaware of the harm or discomfort he's causing. Maybe it's hard for the person to make a quick decision; maybe he hasn't learned good judgment. Research has shown that aggressive, risky drivers are not as well adjusted psychologically as calmer drivers. They tend to be more hostile, depressed, and anxious. So rather than taking offense and trying to retaliate, try thinking, "I wish I could fix things for you. In the meantime, I'll choose not to magnify your pain."

Pretend the other driver is a loved one or neighbor. Think, "We're on the same team (the human team). He's struggling and fallible just like me. He has as much right to be here as I do."

Table 15.1 lists common road rage distortions and their more rational alternatives.

Table 15.1 Road Rage Distortions and Rational Alternatives

Thought Distortion	Rational Alternative
That jerk cut me off!	Let him win. It beats being maimed.
He gave me the finger. Do you realize what that means!?	It means nothing, unless I assign it meaning.
I can't stand this traffic.	This is not WWII. Nobody is shooting at me. The world won't end if I'm late.
I can't let him get away with that!	I don't have to punish the offender. The world won't melt if I let him go. It beats six months of recovery in a hospital.
He's deliberately trying to disrespect me.	Maybe it's not personal. If it is, why should that bother me? Why should I let his nuttiness ruin my drive?
Get out of the passing lane! My progress shouldn't be impeded.	It would be nice if they were more considerate, but they have a right to the road, too. I don't have to let that make me crazy.

The Do's and Don'ts of Wise Driving

Do

- Be vigilant and on the lookout for aggressive or risky drivers.
- Keep your distance from aggressive or risky drivers.
- Let the police catch and punish aggressive or risky drivers. Call 911 (or #77) on your cell phone to report bad driving.
- Ignore gestures and inconsiderate driving.
- Pull over to the right lane and allow drivers to pass you.
- Say, "Sorry, my fault."
- Shrug off aggression.
- Use high beams and the horn sparingly.

- Allow extra time and drive leisurely.
- Drive compassionately.

Don't

- Swallow the hook of another driver.
- Provoke other drivers.
- Glare or make eye contact.
- Roll down your window and yell.
- Block the passing lane.
- Yell or use obscene gestures.
- Do anything that you wouldn't do face to face.
- Take it upon yourself to punish bad drivers.

Supportive Driving Affirmations

Road rage experts James and Nahl suggest rehearsing these affirmations to reinforce the principles we've discussed so far.[1]

- I enjoy making room to let another car into my lane.

- It makes me happy to slow down so that the other car can merge more easily.

- I'm careful to leave enough following distance because I want to avoid giving the impression that I'm tailgating.

- To be more helpful, I like to signal long before I make a turn or switch lanes.

- To show my appreciation, I wave thanks when a motorist does something nice for me.

- I reward myself when my thoughts about other drivers are forgiving rather than hostile.

- I approach pedestrians very slowly in order not to worry them unnecessarily.

- When it's ambiguous who has the right of way, I wait since it is the polite and safe thing to do.

- In parking lots I avoid being pushy and aggressive to give others more of a chance, in case they need the space more than I do. I tell myself, "Someone's always leaving, so I'll get one soon."

- I make myself care about my passengers when I notice them squirming in fear, and I adjust my driving style to accommodate their comfort level.

- Whenever I feel a negative emotion against someone in traffic, I immediately reject that attitude and substitute positive feelings and thoughts.

- When I'm behind the wheel, I keep reminding myself to maintain awareness of my relation to the overall traffic as a willing (not rebellious) participant.

- I will have a safe, relaxed, and enjoyable drive.[2]

Handling Criticism

Few of us enjoy being criticized. However, because we are human we all have rough edges and, probably, no shortage of critics who will gladly point out what they don't appreciate. Criticism might be valid or invalid. It might be constructive (i.e., given with a genuine desire to lift) or hostile (i.e., given with the intent to simply put someone down). The delivery might be kind, tactful, and respectful; or it might be gauche or contemptuous. Since criticism is a fact of life, it is helpful to be prepared for this potential anger hook.

Prepare Yourself

Prepare mentally by keeping an open mind. A beginner's mind is open to feedback. The person with an expert's mind is not, and so does not grow. You might think, "It's good to listen. It helps me see what I can improve. They could be aware of something that I'm not. So I admit I'm wrong. That's being fair. That's what I expect of others."

Realize that no criticism calls your core worth into question. Either the criticism aims at a valid shortcoming, which is external and correctable, or reflects the troubled state of the critic. Either way you can think, "No matter what you do or say, I am still a worthwhile person." Some people find it helpful to imagine a one-way "love shield." If someone, in effect, says, "I hate you," your shield deflects that from your core, while letting through the message, "I don't hate you. I love you." One mother found this concept particularly helpful when her young boy declared his hate for her. She responded, "I don't hate you. I love you so much." It defused his anger, while modeling two ideas: First, anger arises even among people who love each other; it need not change that feeling of love. Second, criticism doesn't change core worth and needn't unduly upset a person.

Realize your choices. The real power lies not in letting anger get out of control but in recognizing the power to make appropriate choices. You can choose not to react angrily (remember the feelings dial meditation, page 125, and the turtle trick, page 214). You can listen to find out if there is merit to the criticism, and agree or disagree. If the person is loud, you might try speaking in a soft voice, even getting quieter as the other person escalates. If the person becomes unreasonable or abusive, you might insist that the person calm down or you won't talk to her. You could walk away or take a time-out. If the criticism seems fair, you might choose to correct your behavior, think about it for a while, apologize, or do nothing. If it is not fair, you can choose to ignore it and have a tough skin. I smile when I think of the guru who said so sweetly, "What do others think of me? Let them think whatever they want. What does it matter?"

Try to Defuse the Critic's Anger with Empathy

Assuming that the critic is fairly reasonable and not abusive, this approach can often be quite effective.

1. Instead of defending yourself or going on the attack, put your ego on the shelf and listen. Think about this for a moment. When you are angry with someone you care about, you probably are already feeling a little isolated and out of control. Perhaps more than getting your way, you most want to be heard, understood, and

respected. If someone were to argue with you, your anger would probably intensify. This may be the position the critic is in. So let that person take a "mental enema" to get all his or her feelings out. Calmly mirror the opposite of anger. Say silently, "Thanks for helping me improve and work on my criticism skills" and "I'm still worthwhile no matter what comes up." Try to understand what's behind those feelings. Ask yourself: "Why might he/she be feeling that way?" "How would I feel if someone did what I am doing?" "Might he/she be having a bad day, or be mad at something else?" Don't be concerned if the feelings don't seem logical at this point. It may take a while to sort them out.

2. Gently ask questions to show the person that you're listening with respect. ("What did I do to upset you? Could you explain what you mean by 'insensitive'? How often did I do that? Would you help me better understand how that upset you?")

3. Paraphrase to check for understanding. You might say, "So it sounds like you're feeling X, because of Y. Do I have that right?" ("So you're feeling . . ."; "You feel like I care more about my friends than you . . ."; "So you wish we could . . ."). Be a little tentative in your paraphrase and check to see that the other person agrees with it.

4. If the criticism is valid, acknowledge it, find a point of agreement, and express your intent to improve. For example:

- "I see your point. You're saying I wasn't sensitive, and I wasn't very sensitive."
- "There's certainly room for improvement."
- "You're right. I'm sorry. I'm going to correct that."
- "From now on, I'm going to . . ."

5. If you disagree with the criticism, try saying:

- "I'm sorry that happened. I can understand your frustration."
- "That's not quite the way it is. I didn't do that, but maybe I can help you solve the problem by . . . (or let's figure out what we can do about this)."[3]

- "We're after the same thing. Blaming each other won't help. Let's . . ."

6. Remember to try humor to lighten things up.

Be Firm with Unreasonable Critics

Not all critics are reasonable. If critics persist in being loud or abusive, then they fall into the realm of difficult people. The rules change somewhat, in that you might have to treat them as you would a bully. Bullies try to control others because they can't control themselves. They'll continue to press you until you require them to take control of themselves. As Horn[4] notes, don't try to appeal to their good nature if it isn't accessible. Instead, early on try, "How about calming down so we can work at solving this," or "I'll listen better if you'll calmly tell me what you're feeling." If you sense that won't work, say firmly one or more of the following:

- "You won't get away with that here."
- "No one talks to me that way."
- "I won't discuss this any further unless you calm down."
- "Calm down. You'll get nowhere if you're so riled."
- "I want you to tell me what you want without criticizing."
- "I don't talk with people who treat me that way. When you're ready to calm down, we can talk."
- "I'm taking a time-out. I'll come back in a half hour and we can see if we're calm enough to talk."
- "I'll listen to you, but only if you're respectful."

Fried and Fried[5] suggest a direct but friendly way to call bullies on their behavior: "You know, some days I just get into the foulest mood and I start picking on other people even when they haven't done anything to me. Are you having a bad day?" Children, so confronted, will often cry at such empathic statements, revealing the pain underneath the controlling behavior.

For critics who like to use put-downs, Huggins[6] suggests that you can ignore the critic, walk away ("Nice talking to you"), or talk it over:

- "How would you like it if I put you down?"
- "I don't like that."
- "Nobody likes to feel inferior."
- "Are you being mean?"

Discrimination and Prejudice

Discrimination and prejudice are unkind, unfair, and heartbreaking. We wish they did not exist. Yet unenlightened humans throughout history—particularly the most vulnerable ones—have feared people who seemed different. Whites persecuted blacks. Whites also persecuted whites who were different, as have blacks. A student related that her father, who came from India, complained of the discrimination he experienced at the hands of Americans. Yet he forbade his daughter from dating an American.

Like anger, discrimination and prejudice can be found anywhere. The real challenge is to not become embittered by these conditions and to prevent them from developing in ourselves. We can think of no instance where retaliation and bitterness overcame discrimination and prejudice. Perhaps the best way to win over enemies is to make them friends and to earn their respect through excellence, grace, and humor. We have also observed that soldiers who killed with hatred are more likely to be traumatized than soldiers who respected their enemy and fought them only out of a sense of duty.

It is possible to work for fairness without hatred. For example, Martin Luther King, Jr., was impassioned, but he was not hostile. When Malcolm X returned from Mecca, he realized that whites were not all as bad as he'd supposed and blacks were not all as good.

We have already explored some examples of nobility of spirit. For example, Booker T. Washington refused to be degraded by hatred, and George Washington Carver made elevating humans central to his life, rather than hatred. We've mentioned two students who prevented bitterness by remembering that all people truly are equal and that love is stronger than hate. In the WWII prison camps, Viktor Frankl refused to detest all Germans because some were compassionate. Without minimizing the scars inflicted upon innocent children by discrimination and prejudice, we can also acknowledge how blaming and hatred inflame those scars.

Besides being a great stress reducer, humor can also be an effective teacher. The story is told of a woman who hit it big at a Las Vegas slot machine. She put her quarters in a plastic bucket and told her husband she would put the bucket in the hotel room and meet him for dinner. As the elevator opened, she noticed two well-dressed African American men standing inside. One was particularly large. Fighting her urge to stereotype, she decided to overcome her fears and entered the elevator. After the doors closed, one of the men said, "Hit the floor." Petrified, the woman did just that, quarters flying all over her and the floor. As she was lying spread-eagled, one of the men, trying to suppress a laugh, said, "I meant that my friend should hit the button for our floor. Which floor are you going to, ma'am?" The men helped her gather the quarters and escorted her to her room. Through the door she could hear the men bursting into hysterical laughter as they walked away. The next day a bouquet of roses arrived. Attached to each rose was a fifty-dollar bill, and there was a note that said, "Thanks for the best laugh we've had in ages." It was signed: Michael Jordan and Eddie Murphy. While this story, of course, is merely urban legend and has been denied by both celebrities, it reminds us not to judge people by their looks.

Computers, Getting Lost, and Other Frustrations

Hooks such as computer problems and getting lost can also be good tests of our anger management mastery. We know someone who is usually fairly placid—except when he gets lost or his computer inexplicably loses its formatting. Both hooks reflect a loss of control that is exacerbated by an overly tight schedule that is somewhat imbalanced. He'll report with some embarrassment, "I have this conversation with my computer, as though there is a little man inside who is deliberately causing me many hours of extra work." Quite humorously, the anger management strategy that seemed to work the best was forgiving that "little man." "Since my screaming didn't seem to resolve the program's design flaw, I decided to just accept the glitch until I can afford to replace the software." Other steps, which are really a summary of some of the skill's we've previously explored, include thinking:

- "Calm down. It isn't worth losing my peace and going crazy over this."
- "I'll think much more rationally if I stay calm."
- "It's okay if I don't always get what I want."
- "Sometimes things like this just happen. That's part of life."
- "I can really handle this. It will pass, and it probably won't be such a big deal in a few days or weeks."
- "If nothing seems to be helping, perhaps the best thing to do is take a break and do something else."
- "Maybe this experience can somehow benefit others."
- "Take two easy, deep breaths and connect with my image of core worth or constructive power."
- "Maybe there's a source of help I've overlooked."
- "This loss of control is temporary and limited. It won't spill over into other areas of my life."

Defusing Frustration: The Fast-Forward Technique

When a frustrating or upsetting event confronts us, we often get mired or stuck in it, obsessing and preoccupying in the angry image, thinking, "I hate this. I can't stand this." The very words make the situation more disagreeable and arousing. The antidote is to "fast-forward" past this upsetting stuck point.

1. Say to yourself, "I can handle this." These words are calming.

2. Replace complaining (which makes you powerless) with action. Complaining is just a way to keep things as they are—it makes us feel like helpless victims. Ask, "Is there something that I could do to remedy this?" If there is, do it quickly and bypass the anger.

3. Fast-forward past "why." Often, asking "Why is this happening?" is not really seeking an answer but is just whining and expressing resentment ("I don't want it to be this way! I won't accept this."). The answer to this question is because the world and everybody in it are imperfect. Change the question to, "Is it possible to figure out the cause of this frustration and do something to remedy it?" If so, take action; if not, move on to step 4.

4. Instead of raging, "I can't accept this," think, "Bad days happen—that's life. This, too, will pass." Some days simply don't go well.

5. See yourself on the other side of the angry situation. Fast-forward to the next evening, at home relaxing. Perhaps you have solved the problem. Perhaps you have accepted life's imperfections and the fact that improvements are often slow to take place. Perhaps you can see yourself on vacation, seeing this situation in perspective as but a glitch in life, and leaving it back at the office.

6. Ask yourself, "Am I so upset because I am overlooking some deeper needs? Would I be happier with more rest, downtime, paying attention to what's bothering me?" Resolve to get through this upsetting moment and then pay attention to those things. Perhaps work this out in your journal.

Drills

- Drive in the right-hand lane. Relax. Enjoy the ride. Enjoy the time to reflect.
- Look for ways to be kind to other drivers.
- Leave earlier than usual. Allow time for delays.
- Practice your calming down skills while delayed, criticized, or frustrated (easy, deep breaths, the turtle trick, HEALS, etc.).
- Practice saying, "Maybe I'm wrong."

Reflections

Nothing is so vulgar as to always be in a hurry.
(Oliver Wendell Holmes)

If we are willing to look at another person's behavior toward us as a reflection of the state of their relationship with themselves rather than as a statement about our value as a person, then we will, over a period of time, cease to react at all.
(Anonymous)

How we react to criticism and mistreatment is a major determinant of our peace of mind.
(Anonymous)

Don't confuse aggression and violence with strength.
(Anonymous)

Suggested Activity

Try the fast-forward technique the next time you are in traffic, criticized, or frustrated.

16

Caring for the Soul

Thou wilt keep him in perfect peace whose mind is stayed on thee.

Isa. 26:3

WE MIGHT REGARD problem anger as a symptom, a warning that something is wrong inside. Sometimes the warning signals a lack of spiritual peace or balance.

Studies of children have found that aggressive behavior is predicted by their feeling miserable or depressed, having a negative self-image, feeling disconnected from other children, and seeing others win conflict by violence. Aggressive children were also less likely to regularly worship.[1] We might, then, more accurately view bullies as unhappy rather than overconfident or innately mean.

Although Freud and Ellis attributed neurotic guilt to religion, the research paints a different picture.[2] In adults, the religiously committed are less stressed, less depressed, less likely to commit suicide, less likely to abuse drugs, and are more satisfied with life and marriage. They live longer, with lower rates of high blood pressure and other diseases. In short, the preponderance of evidence suggests that religious commitment is associated with better mental, physical, and social health. Such benefits are not predicted by religious affiliation or denomination (e.g., Methodist, Muslim, Jew), but by the depth of one's faith—the degree to which individuals live their faith. In the research, religious commitment is typically operationalized as attendance at a church/synagogue/mosque/temple, prayer, and reading sacred works. It also includes a relationship with God, making beliefs an important part of one's life, and connecting with others in the religious community.

Why Is Religious Commitment Beneficial?

While the statistics do not explain the reasons why, we might surmise why the so-called "faith factor" is associated with positive health outcomes, especially as relates to our exploration of problem anger.

1. Self-esteem is heightened by knowing that one is infinitely loved, infinitely worthwhile, and unlimited in potential. In one study, high self-esteem was associated with viewing God as loving.[3] It is easier to let the negative opinions or offenses of others roll off one's back when one knows that one's value is rooted in deeper, more spiritual truths.

2. In their unadulterated forms, all the major world religions teach values that are inconsistent with problem anger: patience, tolerance, forgiveness, kindness, compassion, etc. "Love thy neighbor as thyself" is found in similar words across diverse religious traditions. I'm thankful for the WWII officer who told me when on retreat, "Pray in advance for love for those people you'll one day lead." I found that to be a very effective approach to leadership.

3. Religious beliefs provide a larger perspective—a sense of meaning, purpose, peace, and hope that is greater than the chaos of everyday living. All the major world religions teach a sense of continuity beyond this life. Such an eternal view helps to put temporary irritations in perspective. It also reminds us that all things cannot be completed in this life, but the godly life eventually leads to all good outcomes—removing much pressure. Meaning is encouraged through

selfless service, so we stop seeing the world purely in terms of pleasure and needs.

4. The larger view helps one to place control in perspective. Individuals realize that they can strive to control themselves and be an influence for much good, but there is a grander force piloting the world. Thus, we can release control when it is warranted. This is the basis of the Serenity Prayer used by Alcoholics Anonymous, generally attributed to theologian Reinhold Niebuhr:[4]

> *God, grant me the serenity to*
> *accept the things I cannot change,*
> *courage to change the things I can;*
> *and wisdom to know the difference.*
>
> *Living one day at a time,*
> *enjoying one moment at a time;*
> *accepting hardship as a pathway to peace;*
> *taking, as He did, this sinful world*
> *as it is, not as I would have it;*
>
> *Trusting that You will make all things*
> *right if I surrender to Your will;*
> *So that I may be reasonably happy in this life*
> *and supremely happy with You forever in the next.*
> *Amen.*

Or as Martin Luther King, Jr., said, "My obligation is to do the right thing. The rest is in God's hands."

5. Peace of conscience is encouraged by adhering to universally valued moral principles, including honesty, fairness, fidelity, and schooling of the appetites.

6. Religion affords a sense of connection. Religion derives from the Latin word *religare*, which means "to bind together." Religious communities support their members in diverse ways. Members of the communities can support one another in living ethical lives, despite the pressures of the world. They come together for important rituals to help each other grieve, celebrate, and worship— reminding each other that they are part of God's family. One teenager said, "Church is a time to be friendly with people of all ages. I feel more secure with God, a part of God's family. Church makes my relationship with God stronger—it helps me think of God more; it's like having another friend." Members of a religious community can provide emotional and temporal support in times of need. In such times, many people turn to pastoral counselors, who can augment psychological counseling with spiritual support. Religion also promotes connection and a sense of communion with one's creator. Said one, "I feel a great sense of comfort as I draw close to God through prayer."

7. Religion provides a way to reconcile with God and start anew. Generally, the method involves acknowledging errors, making amends, and striving to forsake the offensive behaviors.

8. Whether it is observed on Friday, Saturday, or Sunday, the Sabbath provides a physical and emotional rest from the cares of the world and a chance for renewal of the spirit.

9. Most religions advise members to take care of the body, through proper rest, nutrition, and physical activity. They also exhort individuals to solidify the family and respect its members.

Religion or Spirituality?

Thomas Moore has written:

> For good reason we go to church, temple, or mosque regularly and at appointed times: it's easy for consciousness to become lodged in the material world and to forget the spiritual. Sacred technology is largely

aimed at helping us remain conscious of spiritual ideas and values . . . There are two ways of thinking about church and religion. One is that we go to church in order to be in the presence of the holy, to learn and to have our lives influenced by that presence. The other is that church teaches us directly and symbolically to see the sacred dimension of everyday life.[5]

The word *spirituality* derives from the Latin root *spiritus*, meaning "breath," referring to the breath of life. The word suggests experiencing the sacred, divine, and holy with reverence, gratitude, awe, devotion, humility, and communion. *Religion* derives both from *religare* (binding together) and *religio*, meaning holiness and reverence for divinity. The roots suggest an image of people coming together to promote spirituality.

Undefiled religion can promote deep and rich spirituality. In their pure forms, religion and spirituality complement each other. Thus, Mother Teresa, Albert Schweitzer, the Dalai Lama, and other great humanitarians have been both spiritual and religious.

Perhaps understandably, some people abandon religion because of disappointments or hurts. Maybe it was hypocrisy or excesses among those who "should know better." Perhaps it was disappointment in themselves. Since humans will always be fallible, the view of a church/temple/mosque as a "hospital for the sinner" can sometimes help us view shortfalls more compassionately.[6] Religion does not guarantee perfection in people or a life free of suffering. However, religion affords hope that people might improve, help in bearing up under suffering, and a sense that there is no final defeat.

Certainly, there are many ways to cultivate religious commitment, including taking the time to read holy writ, pray, worship, reflect, settle on living virtuously, and associate with a religious community. The research suggests that intrinsic spirituality confers the greatest health benefits. This implies that one lives according to his or her beliefs without expectation of personal safety or social acceptance.

Malcolm Muggeridge, a distinguished British author and journalist, nicely summarizes many of the points in this chapter:

I feel so strongly at the end of my life that nothing can happen to us in any circumstances that is not part of God's purpose for us. Therefore, we have nothing to fear, nothing to worry about, except that we should rebel against His purpose, that we should fail to detect it and fail to establish some sort of relationship with Him, and His divine will. On this basis, there can be no black despair, no throwing in of our hand . . . (As one approaches death) you know beyond any shadow of doubt that, as an infinitesimal particle of God's creation, you are a participant in God's purpose for His creation, and that that purpose is loving and not hating, is creative and not destructive, is everlasting and not temporal, is universal and not particular. With this certainty comes an extraordinary sense of comfort and joy. Nothing that happens in this world need shake that feeling; all the happenings in this world, including the most terrible disasters and suffering, will be seen in eternity as in some mysterious way a blessing, as a part of God's love. We ourselves are part of that love.[7]

Reflections

Without prayer, I should have been a lunatic long ago.
(Mohandas Gandhi)

Strive with your whole being to attain perfection.
(Buddha)

The great spiritual practitioners are those who have made a pledge, or developed the determination, to eradicate all of their negative states of mind in order to help to bring the ultimate happiness to all sentient beings.
(Dalai Lama)

We must respect and appreciate the value of all the different major world religious traditions. All of these religions can make an effective contribution for the benefit of humanity. They are all designed to make the individual a happier person, and the world a better place [provided that] the individual practitioner sincerely practice[s] the teachings of that religion.
(Dalai Lama)

Psychology is incomplete if it doesn't include spirituality.

(Thomas Moore)

One thing we know: our God is your God . . . God loves us all . . . No man, be he red man or white, can be apart. We are brothers after all.

(Chief Seattle, 1855)

The vast cosmos of the different forces of nature is tied together by God's directing power. Everything works in mutual harmony with the Divine Plan.

(Paramahansa Yogananda)

When one has realized God, he no longer feels that others are different from himself.

(Paramahansa Yogananda)

Spirit is an essential need of human nature. There is something in all of us that seeks the spiritual . . . Spiritual experience is not taught: it is found, uncovered, and recovered.

(Rachel Naomi Remen, M.D.)

Perfect love casteth out fear.

(1 John 4:18)

As I grew older and learned about different faiths, I came to believe that there was after all but One God with different names: Allah, Tao, the Creator.

(Jane Goodall)

We look at it and we do not see it; Its name is The Invisible.

(Lao Tzu)

Suggested Activities

1. Ponder: Have there been times in your life when you felt spiritual feelings? What might enrich your spiritual life? You might explore this in your journal.

2. Think of the essence of human spirituality: wholesome relationships (inner and outer), character or strong values, meaning and purpose in your life, understanding, and resonating with beauty or nature. Are there areas you might wish to cultivate? What would help you to do so?

3. As you ponder the great distress of terrorism, hold an image of love and decency that is greater than that of evil. That image might be one of a loving God or of loving individuals. You might ponder the idea that no eternal defeat befalls decent individuals.

17

Anticipating Angry
Situations

All things are ready if our minds be so.

—William Shakespeare, *Henry V*

WE'VE COVERED A wide range of skills thus far. In this chapter, you'll put them all together and make a plan for using them to help you through future provocations. In the Harvard Grant Study, which has followed college students since the 1940s, psychiatrist George Vaillant found that mature copers in college were more likely to have better mental, physical, social, and occupational health decades later. One of the hallmarks of the mature copers was their ability to anticipate difficult circumstances and make a plan for coping.

Likewise, you'd be wise to have a plan for confronting the hooks that you'll likely encounter. Anger is a little like a migraine headache. Once the pain starts, it can be too late to prevent the headache. The best time for prevention is well before the headache becomes full blown. In a similar fashion, the best way to manage anger is preventively, before it starts to escalate.

Let's start by reviewing the skills you've learned so far. Then you'll make a plan to apply them to future situations.

Summary of Skills

Table 17.1 summarizes the skills we've explored in this book, the chapters that describe them, and whether they can be used before, during, or after exposure to provocations. As an exercise, fill out the last two columns. First, rate how effective you have found each skill to be on a scale of 1 to 10, with 10 meaning extremely effective. Then check those skills that you want to keep in your anger management toolbox to use again.

Table 17.1 Summary of Skills

Anger Management Skill	Chapter	Use			Rate Effective-ness	Want to Use Again (✓)
		Before	During	After		
Calm Breathing; Easy, Deep Breaths	3	•	•	•		
Progressive Muscle Relaxation	3	•		•		
Daily Thought Record; Question-and-Answer Technique	4			•		
Rational Emotive Imagery	4			•		
"Nevertheless" Skills	5	•	•	•		
Rehearsing Strengths	5	•				
Basic Meditation	6	•				
Inner Strength and Self-Soothing Meditation	7	•				
Constructive Power Meditation	7	•				
Core Worth Meditation	7	•				
Confronting Wounds Meditation	7	•		•		
Feelings Dial Meditation	7	•		•		
Wise Warrior Meditation	7	•		•		

Anger Management Skill	Chapter	Use			Rate Effective- ness	Want to Use Again (✓)
		Before	During	After		
Confiding Hidden Wounds in Writing	8			•		
Time Tripping	8			•		
Physical Conditioning	9	•				
Pleasant Activities Scheduling	9	•				
Anger Journal	9	•		•		
Pleasant Imagery Recall	9	•		•		
Time Management/ Organization	9	•				
Loving Moral Inventory	10	•				
Hostility Reduction	11	•				
Forgiving	12		•	•		
Gestalt Chairs Technique	12			•		
Letter of Apology	12			•		
Forgiving in Writing	12			•		
Forgiveness Imagery	12			•		
Speaker–Listener Technique	13		•			
Planning Couples Fun	13	•				
Couples/Family Meeting	13	•		•		
Parent/Child Interviews	13	•				
HEALS	14		•	•		
ASSIST	14		•			
Humor	14		•			
Affirmations	14	•				
Road Rage Strategies/ Supportive Driving Affirmations	15	•	•			
Defusing Criticism with Empathy	15		•			
Fast-Forward Technique for Defusing Frustration	15		•			
Caring for the Soul	16	•	•	•		

Self-Instruction

This exercise derives from the work of well-known psychologist Donald Meichenbaum.[1] It challenges you to prepare for a hook(s) by practicing what you will think and do before, during, and after you encounter the hook.

Think of a hook that you are likely to encounter in the future.

Step 1: Put a check beside each statement that would have meaning for you if chosen as part of your coping repertoire relative to the anticipated hook(s).

Before

☐ I'm going to stay calm so I can function coolly.

☐ I am in control of my anger.

☐ Don't take it personally.

☐ I can win by ignoring, talking it over calmly, or walking away.

☐ I choose whom I let under my skin.

☐ This won't get under my skin unless I let it.

☐ It's not worth getting all upset over.

☐ I'm calm, as if I were in a hot tub.

☐ This is like the dentist. It will be over soon.

☐ Keep your sense of humor.

☐ I've got a plan. I know how to handle this.

☐ I can figure out the best skills to use.

☐ If I find myself getting hot under the collar, I'll know what to do.

☐ I'll figure out what to say.

- ☐ Expect that others will have their own opinions and will disagree with me.

- ☐ I'm responsible for my anger, no one else.

- ☐ People are always fallible, never perfect.

- ☐ Expect this to be difficult. Go slow.

- ☐ I don't have to be perfect to do well.

  Others; specify:

- ☐ _____

- ☐ _____

During

- ☐ Arousal is a signal to calm down and think about what is the best thing to do.

- ☐ Take some easy, deep breaths.

- ☐ Focus on the issues.

- ☐ I don't have to get upset just because the other person is.

- ☐ Be calm. Yelling won't help.

- ☐ This isn't a catastrophe. I'm okay.

- ☐ In the grand scheme of things, this isn't so important.

- ☐ This is hard. I've done well to put up with it so far.

- ☐ It isn't worth it to get angry.

- ☐ I can hold my ground without getting hot.

- ☐ Remove the ego and stay task oriented.

- ☐ The other person is probably hurting and insecure and is not inept on purpose.

- ☐ It's silly to expect things to go my way at all times.

☐ I'll model calmness and maybe calm the other person down.

☐ Problem solve. What's the best thing to do or say now?

☐ Don't assume the worst. Make the best of this.

☐ Try to see the other person's viewpoint.

☐ Remember to try to compromise or negotiate.

☐ There's time to think. This is not a life or death situation.

☐ Remember, I have lots of options. I can go (leave or take a time-out) or stay (ignore the person or try to work this out).

☐ It's okay if everyone doesn't always approve of me.

☐ I can turn down the anger dial.

☐ Keep a light touch (humor?).

☐ Try to be helpful, not defensive.

Others; specify:

☐ _____

☐ _____

After

If the situation is resolved and/or you stayed relatively calm

☐ Good job. I'm getting better at staying calm.

☐ That was a tough one. I did well.

☐ I got upset, but not out of control. I'm doing better.

☐ All in all, not bad. Not bad at all.

☐ I batted about .900 on this one.

☐ It felt good to prepare and succeed.

Others; specify:

☐ _____

☐ _____

After

If the situation wasn't resolved and/or you became angry

☐ This was a tough one, especially because . . . (we were tired and under stress, we don't know how to solve this yet, it was hot, etc.).

☐ I did my best. That's all I can do.

☐ I batted .400. That's not zero.

☐ It's okay. This is difficult, and I'm still learning.

☐ Next time I'll try to do a better job of staying calm. I'll take a break when I start getting hot or take some deep breaths.

☐ It's water under the bridge. Let it go and think about what you'll do tomorrow.

☐ I'll learn from this.

☐ The world probably won't end.

☐ Everyone has setbacks.

☐ Lots of people do poorly but then improve later.

☐ I'll focus on doing my best next time. I'll probably do better.

☐ Big deal. So I messed up. This too will pass.

☐ Will this really matter a year from now?

☐ This is annoying, but not tragic.

☐ I still trust and like myself.

☐ Even though . . . nevertheless.

☐ Instead of pouting, blaming, or getting sore, I'll figure out the next best thing to do.

☐ Even loved ones will disappoint me sometimes.

☐ My downfall isn't the end of me.

☐ Keep trying until you get the hang of it.

☐ You don't always get what you want.

☐ People won't always see things my way.

☐ I have the right to correct my course.

☐ Okay, I botched that. Try again.

☐ I made a mistake. I am not a mistake.

☐ I'm not a failure if I keep trying.

☐ I can't possibly control everything.

☐ I can forgive the other person's shortcomings, bad behavior, etc.

☐ Next time, my plan to stay calm is:

_____

_____

Others; specify:

☐ _____

☐ _____

Step 2: Below, write fifteen statements you would most like to remember to tell yourself before, during, and after you confront the hook(s)—five for before, five for during, and five for after. The statements may come from the above list or you might think of new ones to add.

Before

1. _____

2. _____

3. _____

4. _____

5. _____

During

1. _____

2. _____

3. _____

4. _____

5. _____

After

1. _____

2. _____

3. _____

4. _____

5. _____

Spend a few minutes each day for the next three days mentally rehearsing these statements so that they will be automatic when you need them.

Desensitization

Systematic desensitization is 90 percent effective in reducing anxiety. It is also very effective for calming the sensitized nervous systems of angry people. Essentially, in desensitization we break down a difficult hook into parts, and then pair each part with calm thoughts, feelings, behaviors, and/or physical reactions. With repeated practice the various parts of the hook cease to elicit an anger response. Instead the hook tends to elicit the preferred responses that we've rehearsed.

Take one of your hooks that you have encountered and are likely to encounter again. Build a hierarchy, or a list of aspects of the hook that occur before, during, and after the actual exposure. For example, if driving to work during rush hour is one of your greatest hooks, you might create a list that looks like this:

- Thinking about driving to work the night before
- Picking up my car keys as I leave the house
- Entering the car
- Starting the car
- Driving through town
- Merging into the interstate
- Stop-and-go traffic
- People who cut in front of me when I'm trying to keep a safe distance from cars in front of me
- Noticing my body's arousal
- Drivers passing on the shoulder
- Looking at my watch and realizing I'm going to be late
- People sitting on their horns when I don't close the gap between cars fast enough
- Leaving the interstate
- Battling congestion near the office
- Parking the car
- Getting to my office, thinking about the aggravations of rush hour

Basic desensitization pairs each step on the hierarchy with relaxation, which is incompatible with anger's arousal. It works like this.

1. Begin by finding a quiet place where you can relax and practice for about an hour. Perform progressive muscle relaxation for a few minutes until you are deeply relaxed.

2. Start with the first step on your hierarchy. Think of it for a few seconds, allowing yourself to feel the normal levels of arousal.

3. Then deeply relax. Take two easy, deep breaths and repeat your calming word or phrase. Breathe abdominally, normally. Tense and relax various muscle groups until you feel relaxed. Stay relaxed for a few moments, up to about a minute.

4. Think again of the first step on the hierarchy for a few seconds, again feeling the arousal that occurs. Then take two easy, deep breaths, breathe abdominally, and tense and relax your muscles until you again feel relaxed. Stay relaxed for a few moments, about a minute.

5. Repeat step 4 one more time, and perhaps more if needed, until you can get very relaxed fairly quickly and easily after thinking about this step on your hierarchy.

6. Repeat steps 2 to 5 for the next step on your hierarchy.

7. Continue down the hierarchy in this way for no more than one hour.

8. If at any step on the hierarchy you find it difficult to relax, try going more slowly or adding more progressive muscle relaxation. If it is still difficult to relax, add additional steps before the step you're stuck on and/or break up that step into smaller increments.

9. The following day, pick up by repeating step 1 for the step on your hierarchy that you left off at the previous day. If you can still relax comfortably after thinking about it, proceed down the hierarchy from that point in the same manner as you did before. If needed,

back up until you find a step where relaxation is fairly easy and quick after thinking about it.

10. Keep repeating these procedures until you have worked through all the steps on the hierarchy while maintaining a feeling of relaxation.

What this exercise does is to condition you to respond to each step on the hierarchy with relaxation rather than arousal. With practice, the desired reaction becomes automatic in much the same way that Pavlov conditioned dogs to salivate when he rang a bell.

Variations of Desensitization

Basic desensitization can be augmented by adding other anger management skills. People tend to do this almost instinctively as they relax themselves at each step. The basic desensitization technique can be modified in various creative and effective ways. Each step on your hierarchy can be paired with:

• *Rational thoughts*. At each step see yourself becoming aroused. Identify the irrational thoughts or distortions that are going through your mind. Then see yourself calming down and notice the new thoughts that you are choosing.

• *Coping imagery*. See yourself becoming aroused at each step on the hierarchy. Then see yourself calming yourself down and behaving in calm and reasoned ways.

• *Humor*. If you can, see yourself responding to each step with humor, which replaces angry feelings with feelings of mastery and self-acceptance.

• *Competency imagery*. Make a list of the times in your life when you really felt capable and satisfied with your performance. Pick one and recall it in vivid detail. Then transpose this image and the attendant feelings onto each step of your hierarchy. This is powerful because the image is already part of your personal experience.

- *Creative combinations*. You might pair each step with some uniquely personal combination of relaxation, calming thoughts (e.g., "I'm calm and amused by this"), feelings or images of competence, and/or coping imagery.

Drill

Wrap yourself in an invisible serenity shield prior to a difficult encounter. The shield keeps harm out, keeps peace in, and lets love and concern go through.

Reflections

Battles are won before they are fought.

(Anonymous)

Lapses are normal and don't negate progress.

(Anonymous)

Once we accept things (people, self, situations) as they are, then we are open to seeing what new, creative approaches are called for.

(Anonymous)

Suggested Activities

1. As a quick review, complete the "Summary of Skills" list.
2. After completing the Self-Instruction exercise, rehearse your favorite before, during, and after statements.
3. Create a desensitization hierarchy for an anticipated hook. Work through the hierarchy, first with progressive muscle relaxation, then using rational thoughts, coping imagery, humor, competency imagery, and/or some creative combination of these.

Epilogue

HAVING WORKED YOUR way through this book, you are now well equipped with an array of skills to help you effectively manage anger throughout life. But life is difficult. Who ever learns something once and for all? Some of these skills may have come easily. Others might require deliberate and repeated practice to master. Once skills have been acquired, don't be too surprised if you need to return to this book to reinforce your learning.

Try the best that you know how (which is all anyone can do), be as patient and compassionate as you can, and don't be too hard on the shortcomings of people—including yourself. Focus more on the process and not so much on the outcome, since our lives are works in progress. And realize that there are many other resources to help you when you need or want them (see Appendix B).

To summarize and reinforce the most important ideas and skills, as well as to serve as a quick reminder during stressful times, please review the entire book and list below those ideas and skills that you most want to remember.

1. The ideas or principles that have had the most meaning to me are . . .

_____

_____

_____

_____

2. The skills that I think have the greatest potential for me are . . .

_____

_____

_____

_____

3. The skills that I want to practice more are . . . (Make a plan and take the time to practice these.)

_____

_____

_____

_____

We wish you less anger. More than that, we wish you a calmer, more peaceful journey.

Appendix A

Dietary Guidelines

CHECK TO SEE if your sample menu (see Chapter 9, page 143) meets the following guidelines for healthy eating.

1. Does your plan provide the daily recommended servings from each food group as indicated below? (A person trying to control weight would use the smaller figure for servings.)

Food Group	Servings Recommended Per Day	Examples of One Serving
Breads, cereals, rice, pasta	6 to 11	1 slice of bread 1 ounce ready-to-eat cereal 1/2 bun or bagel 1/2 cup cooked cereal, rice, or pasta
Vegetables	3 to 5	1 cup raw leafy greens 1/2 cup other kinds of vegetables 1/2 cup vegetable juice
Fruits	2 to 4	1 medium apple, banana, or orange 1/2 cup fresh, chopped, cooked, or canned fruit 3/4 cup fruit juice

Food Group	Servings Recommended Per Day	Examples of One Serving
Milk, yogurt and cheese	2 to 3	I cup milk or yogurt (skim or low-fat is best) $1^{1}/2$ ounces natural cheese 2 ounces processed cheese
Meat, poultry, fish, dry beans and peas, eggs, and nuts	2 to 3	Amounts to a total of approximately 6 ounces a day, where I serving is 2 to 3 ounces of cooked lean meat, poultry, or fish. Equivalent to 1 ounce of meat: 1 egg; 2 tablespoons peanut butter; $1/2$ cup cooked dry beans or peas; $1/3$ cup nuts; or $1/2$ cup seeds

2. Does your plan provide variety? That is, do you vary your choices within each group? (Instead of an apple each day, try a banana or strawberries as alternatives.)
3. Does your plan follow the other guidelines presented in Chapter 9?

Appendix B

Resources

Couples and Family Skills

Garcia-Prats, C. M., and J. A. Garcia-Prats. *Good Families Don't Just Happen: What We Learned From Raising Our Ten Sons and How It Can Work For You*. Holbrook, MA: Adams Media Corporation. Principle-based skills, starting with respect between spouses.

Latham, G. I. *The Power of Positive Parenting: A Wonderful Way to Raise Children*. N. Logan, UT: P&T Ink. Useful and thorough guide to steady, consistent, and peaceful parenting.

Lundberg, G., and J. Lundberg. *I Don't Have to Make Everything All Better*. New York: Viking Penguin. A treasure chest of methods for relating to people. Learn how to walk alongside people emotionally, rather than arguing or criticizing.

———. *Married for Better, Not Worse: The Fourteen Secrets to a Happy Marriage*. New York: Viking Penguin. Another down-to-earth treasure for creating a satisfying marriage.

Hendrix, H. *Getting the Love You Want: A Guide for Couples*. New York: HarperPerrenial. Marriage communication skills.

Markman, H., S. Stanley, and S. L. Blumberg. *Fighting* for *Your Marriage: Positive Steps for Preventing Divorce and Preserving a Lasting Love*. San Francisco: Jossey-Bass. From conflict resolution to increasing fun. Practical. Based on solid research.

National Institute of Relationship Enhancement. 12500 Blake Road, Silver Spring, MD 20904 (1-800-THE-NIRE). Well-researched skills training for strengthening couples and family relationships; includes improving communication and conflict resolution. First developed as therapy, now also used for prevention of distress and for marital and premarital enrichment. Practical weekend relationship enhancement seminars. Therapist training. Manuals and tapes for parenting and couples skills. Referrals to NIRE-trained counselors.

Prevention and Relationship Enhancement Program: Resources for a Loving Relationship. P.O. Box 102530, Denver, CO 80250-2530 (1-800-366-0166; www.prepinc.com). *Fighting* for *Your Marriage* and other books. Four excellent, affordable videos help develop communication skills, solve problems, and promote intimacy. Well-researched and respected, PREP is not therapy but is educational and preventive in nature. Includes self-taught programs, workshops, and coached programs.

Antidotes to Stress

Ashe, A. *Days of Grace: A Memoir*. New York: Ballantine. Retaining inner peace and optimism despite tragedy.

Dalai Lama and H. C. Cutler. *The Art of Happiness: A Handbook for Living*. New York: Riverhead. Profound insights on self-esteem and compassion.

Frankl, V. *Man's Search for Meaning*. Boston: Beacon. The classic work on discovering meaning in one's life out of suffering. Written by the Holocaust survivor who founded logotherapy.

Geisel, Theodor. *Oh, the Places You'll Go*. New York: Random House. Part of the Dr. Seuss series; a clever, humorous treatise on human growth and fallibility. Definitely not just for kids.

Hanh, T. N. *Peace Is Every Step*. New York: Bantam. Peaceful monk's practical ways to cultivate inner peace, joy, serenity, and balance.

Linehan, M. M. *Skills Training Manual for Treating Borderline Personality Disorder*. New York: Guilford. Specific skills that are useful for functioning populations as well, including mindfulness, interpersonal effectiveness skills, emotion regulation skills, and distress tolerance skills.

Morgenstern, J. *Organizing from the Inside Out*. New York: Henry Holt. Reduce stress at home or at work by organizing, beautifying, and developing a retrieval system.

Schiraldi, G. R. *Conquer Anxiety, Worry and Nervous Fatigue: A Guide to Greater Peace*. Ellicott City, MD: Chevron. From hyperventilation to worrisome thoughts. "The best book for anxiety we've ever seen." (Sidran Foundation) Contact Chevron Publishing Corp. at 5018 Dorsey Hall Dr., Suite 104, Ellicott City, MD 21042, (410) 740-0065.

————. *Facts to Relax By: A Guide to Relaxation and Stress Reduction*. Provo, UT: Utah Valley Regional Medical Center. A wide range of strategies and resources. Contact Chevron Publishing Corp. at 5018 Dorsey Hall Dr., Suite 104, Ellicott City, MD 21042, (410) 740-0065.

————. *Hope and Help for Depression: A Practical Guide*. Ellicott City, MD: Chevron. Diverse instructions for self-managed treatments and how to find professional help. Contact Chevron Publishing Corp. at 5018 Dorsey Hall Dr., Suite 104, Ellicott City, MD 21042, (410) 740-0065.

————. *The Post-Traumatic Stress Disorder Sourcebook: A Guide to Healing, Recovery and Growth*. Los Angeles: Lowell House. Covers diverse approaches to managing traumatic stress, including anger management. "The most valuable, user-friendly manual on PTSD I have ever seen. Must reading for victims, their families, and their therapists." (Dr. George Everly, Executive Editor, *International Journal of Emergency Mental Health*)

Specifically for Anger

Bramson, R. *Coping with Difficult People*. Garden City, NY: Doubleday. Beyond assertiveness.

Dalai Lama. *Healing Anger: The Power of Patience from a Buddhist Perspective*. Ithaca, NY: Snow Lion. A kind exploration that is mostly consistent with and respectful of other perspectives.

Fried, S., and P. Fried. *Bullies and Victims: Helping Your Child Survive the Schoolyard Battlefield*. New York: M. Evans. Many practical ideas, plus an excellent resource list.

Larson, J., with C. Rodriguez. *Road Rage to Road-Wise*. New York: Tom Doherty. Perhaps the most useful book on road rage.

Schiraldi, G. R. *The Self-Esteem Workbook*. Oakland, CA: New Harbinger. Gets to the core of much problem anger. Based on the successful "Stress and the Healthy Mind" course, University of Maryland. Many effective skills.

Simon, S., and S. Simon. *Forgiveness: How to Make Peace with Your Past and Get on with Your Life*. New York: Warner. When unhealed and unresolved hurts affect your present mood and functioning.

Professional Books

Beck, A. T. *Prisoners of Hate: The Cognitive Basis of Anger, Hostility, and Violence*. New York: HarperCollins. A scholarly exploration of anger—its causes and manifestations.

Kassinove, H., ed. *Anger Disorders: Definition, Diagnosis, and Treatment*. Washington, DC: Taylor and Francis. Explores the nature of anger, including what it is and how it arises, when it is disordered, how it is measured and treated, and criminality and cross-cultural considerations.

Referrals: Finding Mental Health Professionals

Alliance for Children and Families. 11700 West Lake Park Dr., Milwaukee, WI 5322 (414-359-1040). Referrals to family/social service agencies, which accept payments on a sliding scale.

American Academy of Child and Adolescent Psychiatry. 3615 Wisconsin Ave., NW., Washington, DC 20016 (202-966-7300; 1-800-333-7636). Call or write for referral information about child and adolescent psychiatrists in your area.

American Association for Marriage and Family Therapy. 1133 Fifteenth St., NW, Suite 300, ATTN: Referrals, Washington, DC 20005 (202-452-0109). Marriage and family therapists.

American Association of Pastoral Counselors. 9504A Lee Highway, Fairfax, VA 22031 (703-385-6967). Many who seek help in times of need turn first to a clergy person. This association provides referrals to certified pastoral counselors who consider both spiritual and psychological needs.

American Professional Society on the Abuse of Children (APSAC), PO Box 26901, CHO 3B-3406, Oklahoma City, OK 73190 (405-271-8202). Refers children and adults to various resources through state chapters.

American Psychiatric Association. 1400 K St., NW, Washington, DC 20005 (202-682-6220). Call or write the Public Affairs office for referrals to psychiatrists in your area.

American Psychological Association. 750 First St., NE, Washington DC 20002 (202-336-5500 or 5800; 1-800-374-2721). Call or write for referrals to psychologists in your area.

Association for Advancement of Behavior Therapy. 305 7th Ave., New York, NY 10001 (212-647-1890; 1-800-685-AABT). Provides a membership listing, including specialty areas, of mental health professionals focusing on behavior therapy and cognitive behavior therapy in your state, along with a complimentary brochure, "Guidelines for Choosing a Behavior Therapist."

Center for Mental Health Services, Knowledge Exchange Network. P.O. Box 4290, Washington, DC 20015 (1-800-789-2647). Referrals to local community mental health centers and family service agencies, both of which provide mental services on a sliding fee scale. Also information on mental health agencies, support groups, and clearinghouses.

Childhelp USA. 15757 N. 78 St., Scottsdale, AZ 85260 (1-800-422-4453). In addition to referrals to therapists, crisis centers, and child protective services, hot line also provides crisis counseling for children, troubled parents, and adult survivors. Free literature on child abuse, parenting, and recovery.

EMDR Institute. P.O. Box 51010, Pacific Grove, CA 93950 (831-372-3900 ext. 16; 1-800-780-3637). Referrals for clinicians trained in eye movement densensitization and reprocessing (EMDR), which can also help to resolve anger from deep or traumatic offenses.

National Association of Social Workers. 750 First St., NE, Suite 700, Washington, DC 20002-4241 (202-408-8600; 1-800-638-8799). Referrals to qualified clinical social workers in your area.

National Board for Certified Counselors. 3 Terrace Way, Suite D, Greensboro, NC 27403 (336-547-0607). Referrals for certified clinical mental health counselors.

National Mental Health Association. 1021 Prince St., Alexandria, VA 22314-2971 (703-684-7722; 1-800-969-NMHA). Provides list of affiliate mental health organizations in your area that can provide resources and information about self-help groups, treatment professionals, and community clinics.

TIR Association. 13 NW Barry Rd., Suite 214, Kansas City, MO 64155-2728 (816-468-4945). Referrals to clinicians offering traumatic incident reduction (TIR), which can sometimes help to resolve anger from deep or traumatic offenses.

Organizations and Services: Prevention

Compassion Power. 16220 Frederick Rd., Suite 404, Gaithersburg, MD 20877 (301-921-2010). Offers a wide range of educational–therapeutic programs, books, and tapes to manage anger, improve mental health, and improve interpersonal relationships.

Martial Arts for Peace Association. P.O. Box 816, Middlebury, VT 05753 (1-800-848-6021). Helps children learn how to avoid violence and stand up to abusers in nonviolent ways. Beautiful publications.

Sopris West. 4093 Specialty Place, Longmont, CO 80504 (303-651-2829; 1-800-547-6747). Diverse resources to help parents and teachers help children. Includes "Helping Kids Handle . . ." Series (Anger, Put-Downs, Conflict), and handling "tough kids" series.

The STOP Violence Coalition of Kansas City. 301 E. Armour, #440, Kansas City, MO 64111 (816-753-8002). Dedicated to the prevention of interpersonal violence, teaches conflict avoidance, mediation, and resolution. "Kindness is Contagious" and other programs for schools.

Agencies/Organizations/Victim's Services

Check the telephone directory for violence shelters, counseling and support groups for victims and perpetrators, counseling referrals, hot lines, legal services, welfare, referrals to counselors (sliding scale), etc. Look under crisis intervention, domestic violence/abuse information and treatment centers, social services, human services, shelters, women's organizations, or family services.

Childhelp USA. See description Under Referrals section.

Mothers Against Drunk Driving (MADD). 511 E. John Carpenter Fwy, Suite 700, Irving, TX 75062 (1-800-GET-MADD). Victim-to-victim support services include support groups, diverse publications (crash victim, mourning, legal issues, etc.), court accompaniment, help with navigating the criminal justice system, and training.

National Center for Victims of Crime. 2000 M. St., NW, Suite 480, Washington, DC 20036 (1-800-FYI-CALL). Referrals for victims of any violent crime (sexual abuse, domestic violence, stalking, hate crime, etc.) to shelters, support groups, and legal advocacy programs. Also information bulletins on these topics.

National Clearinghouse on Child Abuse and Neglect Information. 330 C St., SW, Washington, DC 20447 (703-385-7565; 1-800-394-3366). General information on all aspects of child mistreatment for the public and professionals.

National Domestic Violence Hotline. (1-800-799-SAFE). Twenty-four-hour hot line with multilingual and deaf capabilities. Serves victims and concerned family and friends. Helps victims with issues of safety, shelter, counseling, and legal advice. Also helps batterers get help. Printed information.

National Organization for Victims Assistance (NOVA). 1730 Park Road NW, Washington, DC 20010 (202-232-6682; 1-800-TRY-NOVA). Support and advocacy for crime victims. Referrals to victim assistance programs (battered women's programs, support groups, rape crisis centers, legal and medical advice, etc.). Crisis Response Team Project formed to deal with community crises. Training and education for helpers.

Prevent Child Abuse America. 200 S. Michigan Ave, 17th Floor, Chicago, IL 60604 (1-800-CHILDREN). Extensive printed material. Healthy Families America is a home visiting service for parents which teaches parenting skills, links parents to resources, and provides a helping hand.

Survivor and Support Groups

In addition to the following, check your local newspaper, white pages, and library, and with police, hospitals, mental health professionals, and mental health agencies.

American Self-Help Group Clearinghouse. 100 East Hannover Ave., Suite 202, Cedar Knolls, NJ 07927-2020 (973-326-6789; 1-800-367-6274 in NJ.). Directs caller to diverse self-help groups. Inexpensive sourcebook lists national and model self-help groups, guide-lines for forming self-help groups, and other clearinghouses.

National Clearinghouse for Alcohol and Drug Information. (1-800-662-HELP). Referrals to detoxification and rehabilitation programs, as well as alcohol and drug support groups. Various publications on alcohol and substances.

National Mental Health Consumers' Self-Help Clearinghouse. 1211 Chestnut St., Suite 1207, Philadelphia, PA 19107 (1-800-553-4539). Technical assistance for self-help groups, as well as help in locating self-help groups. Also furnishes inexpensive informational packets.

National Self-Help Clearinghouse. c/o CUNY Graduate Center, 365 5th Ave., Suite 3300, New York, NY 10016 (212-817-1822). Directs callers to self-help and support groups. Also trains facilitators.

Below is a sampling of self-help/support groups whose numbers may be obtained from the above clearinghouses/helplines. Many are based on the AA twelve-step model.

Adult Children of Alcoholics.

Al-Anon Family Groups and Alateen. For those whose lives have been affected by the drinking of a family member.

Alcoholics Anonymous.

Cocaine Anonymous.

The Compassionate Friends. Information and referrals to support groups for bereaved parents, siblings, and grandparents who grieve the death of a child.

Gamblers Anonymous.

Incest Survivors Anonymous.

Narcotics Anonymous. Support groups for users.

National Amputation Foundation.

National SHARE Office. St. Joseph Health Center, 300 First Capitol Dr., St. Charles, MO 63301-2893 (636-947-6164; 1-800-821-6819). Support for families who have suffered perinatal loss.

Overeaters Anonymous.

Parents Anonymous. For parents who batter and wish to learn effective parenting. Professionally facilitated and peer led. Not a twelve-step program.

Parents of Murdered Children. Support groups for anyone who has lost someone to homicide. Also court accompaniment, antiviolence advocacy, questions related to unsolved cases of suicide/homicide, training for support groups and sensitivity to violence.

Parents United International and Adults Molested as Children. For sexually abused victims of all ages, offenders, and support persons (spouses, parents, etc.).

Pregnancy and Infant Loss Center. 1421 E. Wayzata Blvd, Suite 70, Wayzata, MN 55391 (952-473-9372). Grief support for miscarriage, stillbirth, and infant death. Resources and education. Referrals to support groups.

Sex Addicts Anonymous.

SIDS Alliance (Sudden Infant Death Syndrome).

Survivors of Incest Anonymous. Also provides a hot line and bimonthly bulletins.

Survivors of Suicide. For families and friends of suicide victims.

Widowed Persons Service. American Association of Retired Persons. Referrals for widows and widowers to information, services, and support programs.

Appendix C

Stress, Anger, and Cardiovascular Disease: A Comprehensive Model

THE MODEL AT the end of this appendix (page 283) details the theoretical relationship between stress, anger, and cardiovascular disease. Stress is often defined as the response of the body to threats or demands. The stress response is called a neuroendocrine response; the brain acts like a conductor and orchestrates a cascade of neural (nerves) and endocrine (hormonal) messages that target various organs. Anger/hostility is thought to be a risk factor for cardiovascular disease because all of the major stress pathways (A to E in the model) are theoretically activated when a person becomes aroused. This model depicts stress as not only a response but also a process that involves continuous interactions and adjustments (transactions) between an individual and the environment. In part, this book is about making those interactions and adjustments as "appropriate" and healthy as possible, thereby enabling a person to become an active agent in his or her well-being rather than a passive victim of the world's unpleasantries.

The upper portion of the model is based on Ellis's A-B-C theory of emotional arousal. The stressor (anger hook) is the *Activating* event. The thoughts or *Beliefs* that follow are influenced by one's self esteem and deeply held core beliefs. Hot thoughts lead to anger (emotional *Consequences*) and subsequent angry behaviors. Certain behaviors can feed back to increase anger and further erode self-esteem.

Thoughts take place in the level of the brain called the neocortex. The nature of the thoughts elicits one's emotions, which are regulated by the brain's limbic system. When angry, a person's brain prepares the body for fight or flight by sending neuroendocrine "commands" through the hypothalamus to the body via various pathways. These commands are adaptive in the short term because they energize a person. In the long run, however, chronic anger may exact a toll on the body.

Certain behavioral and psychophysiological factors, though not depicted in the model, may have a buffering effect on the stress response. These factors include:

- "Good" genes
- Female gender
- Good coping skills
- Hardy personality
- Adequate nutrition, rest, and exercise
- Relaxation skills
- Social support
- Belief in a higher power and worship
- Internal locus of control

In contrast, numerous factors may exacerbate the stress response, including elevated cardiovascular reactivity (being a hot reactor); lack of social support; poor coping skills; male gender; poor diet, exercise, and sleep habits; and genetics (e.g., family history of hypertension and/or other cardiovascular risks).

Model Components

Stressor/Hooks(s): Internal and/or external events that can be acute, episodic, or chronic in nature.

Thoughts: Beliefs and perceptions regarding those events. Distortions, or "hot thoughts," have the potential to increase arousal.

Self-Esteem: A realistic, appreciative opinion of oneself, resulting from unconditional love, worth, and growth.

Research and/or clinical experience support a relationship between low self-esteem and manifestations of physical and mental illness, such as physical and emotional abuse, drug abuse, and the like. The feedback loop in the model suggests that emotional and behavioral states may further erode self-esteem.

Core Belief(s): Underlying beliefs (e.g., people are bad and inept, and shouldn't be; I'm a person, therefore I'm inept) and expectations that may be unrealistic can result in distorted cognitions.

Anger: The emotion resulting from the thoughts.

Behavior(s): Voluntary actions that follow from and influence an individual's emotions. Disproportionate anger may contribute to unhealthy behaviors such as a sedentary lifestyle, poor nutrition, drug abuse, delinquency, and the like.

Hypothalamus: A part of the brain that organizes the "fight or flight" response.

Primary Stress Response Pathways

A represents the immediate pathway—direct innervation of organs by the sympathetic branch (SNS) of the autonomic nervous system. This pathway is the fastest acting pathway, given the capability of nerves to transmit messages rapidly. The immediate effects of direct organ innervation are:

- Increased heart rate, stroke volume, and, therefore, cardiac output
- Vasodilation of the coronary and deep muscle arteries
- Vasoconstriction of blood vessels in the skin, abdominal viscera, and kidneys
- Increased blood coagulation and decreased clotting time
- Increased glycogenolysis, the conversion of stored sugar (glycogen) to glucose
- Increased release of glucose from the liver (raises blood glucose)

- Inhibited digestion
- Increased arterial blood pressure
- Increased metabolic rate
- Increased brain activity
- Increased sweat gland activity
- Dilation of bronchioles in the lungs
- Increased respiration rate and depth
- Dilation of pupils
- Increased skeletal muscle contractility
- Breakdown of fatty tissue, raising blood fatty acid (FFA) levels, triglycerides, and/or cholesterol

B represents the intermediate pathway due to the delayed onset and longer duration of effects. A neuron originates in the spine and terminates in the adrenal medulla. When activated, it stimulates the adrenal medulla to release epinephrine (Epi) and norepinephrine (NE) into the circulation; the longer-acting nature of hormones serves to sustain the stress response. The combined effects of Epi and NE are an increase in blood pressure and cardiac output. The specific effects are:

- Increased heart rate, stroke volume, and cardiac output
- Vasodilation of the coronary arteries
- Increased glycogenolysis
- Increased glucose release from the liver
- Vasoconstriction of peripheral skin arterioles
- Vasoconstriction of superficial muscle arterioles
- Increased blood coagulation and decreased clotting time

The remaining pathways are long-term pathways involving the pituitary, a gland situated just under the hypothalamus. The pituitary is referred to as the "master" endocrine gland, as it controls the activity of other endocrine glands. The anterior pituitary releases trophic hormones (ACTH and TSH) into the bloodstream, which in turn stimulate other endocrine glands (i.e., adrenal cortex and thyroid) to release hormones (i.e., cortisol, aldosterone, thyroxine) into the bloodstream. In turn, these hormones target and excite various tissues and organs (e.g., liver, kidneys, heart, and arterioles).

C represents the ACTH pathway. This is a long-term pathway in which ACTH (adrenocorticotrophic hormone) is released from the anterior pituitary and targets the adrenal cortex. The adrenal cortex responds by releasing glucocorticoids and mineralocorticoids. The chief glucocorticoid is cortisol (Cor), which has numerous, potentially detrimental effects. Those related to cardiovascular disease include:

- Elevated insulin levels and abdominal fat storage
- Mobilization of fatty acids from fat cells
- Increased gluconeogenesis, the liver's formation of glucose from amino acids and other molecules
- Increased blood glucose

Cortisol also decreases the number and/or activity of white blood cells and plays a role in the atrophy of lymphatic structures including the thymus, thereby potentially compromising the immune system. It also acts with Epi to produce anti-inflammatory effects. The chief mineralocorticoid is aldosterone (Ald), which maintains blood sodium homeostasis via increased sodium retention, increased water retention by the kidneys, and increased blood and interstitial fluid volume. Aldosterone also has an inflammatory effect and increases cardiac output.

D represents the thyroxine (Thy) pathway, one of the most significant because of the duration of its effects. Thyroid stimulating hormone (TSH) is released from the anterior pituitary and targets the thyroid, which releases thyroxine. This hormone has numerous physiological effects, many of which are implicated in cardiovascular disease, including:

- Increased metabolic rate via an increase in general metabolism in almost all cells
- Increased (cellular) oxygen consumption
- Increased respiration rate and depth
- Increased heart rate and cardiac output
- Increased peripheral resistance
- In general, an increase in protein catabolism
- Increased internal body temperature
- Increased gastrointestinal motility, absorption, and secretion of digestive juices
- Increased cerebration (i.e., irritability, anxiety, and insomnia)

Regarding the vasopressin pathway, E, the anterior hypothalamus stimulates the posterior pituitary to release the neurotransmitter vasopressin, a potent vasoconstrictor. Its effects result in increased smooth muscle contraction (clamping of the arteries), increased renal permeability to water, water reabsorption, decreased perspiration, increased blood volume, and increased arterial blood pressure. There are several theories that suggest that transient increases in blood pressure may result in sustained hypertension, a form of cardiovascular disease and a primary risk factor for coronary artery disease.

The endothelial injury hypothesis has been proposed to explain the involvement of the various pathways in the development of coronary artery disease, the most prevalent cardiovascular disease. The theory posits that injury to the thin layer of endothelial cells of the arterial wall triggers the initiation of plaque formation. This injury may occur as the result of mechanical forces (i.e., blood pressure increases hemodynamic forces on arterial wall) or via chemical means (i.e., increased LDL-C, catecholamines, corticoids, etc.). Atherosclerosis is the process that entails endothelial injury, plaque formation, lesion development, and subsequent plaque buildup.

Figure C.1 Stress, Anger, and Cardiovascular Disease: A Comprehensive Model

(by Melissa Hallmark Kerr)

Key

Hormones:	TSH:	Thyroid Stimulating Hormone	HDL-C:	High Density Lipoprotein Cholesterol
Glands:	Epi:	Epinephrine		
	NE:	Norepinephrine	FFA:	Free Fatty Acids
Pathways:	Cor:	Cortisol	CVD:	Cardiovascular Disease
	Ald:	Aldosterone		
Neuroendocrine Effects:	Thy:	Thyroxine		
	MAP:	Mean Arterial Pressure (blood pressure)		
ACTH: Adrenocorticotrophic Hormone	LDL-C:	Low Density Lipoprotein Cholesterol		

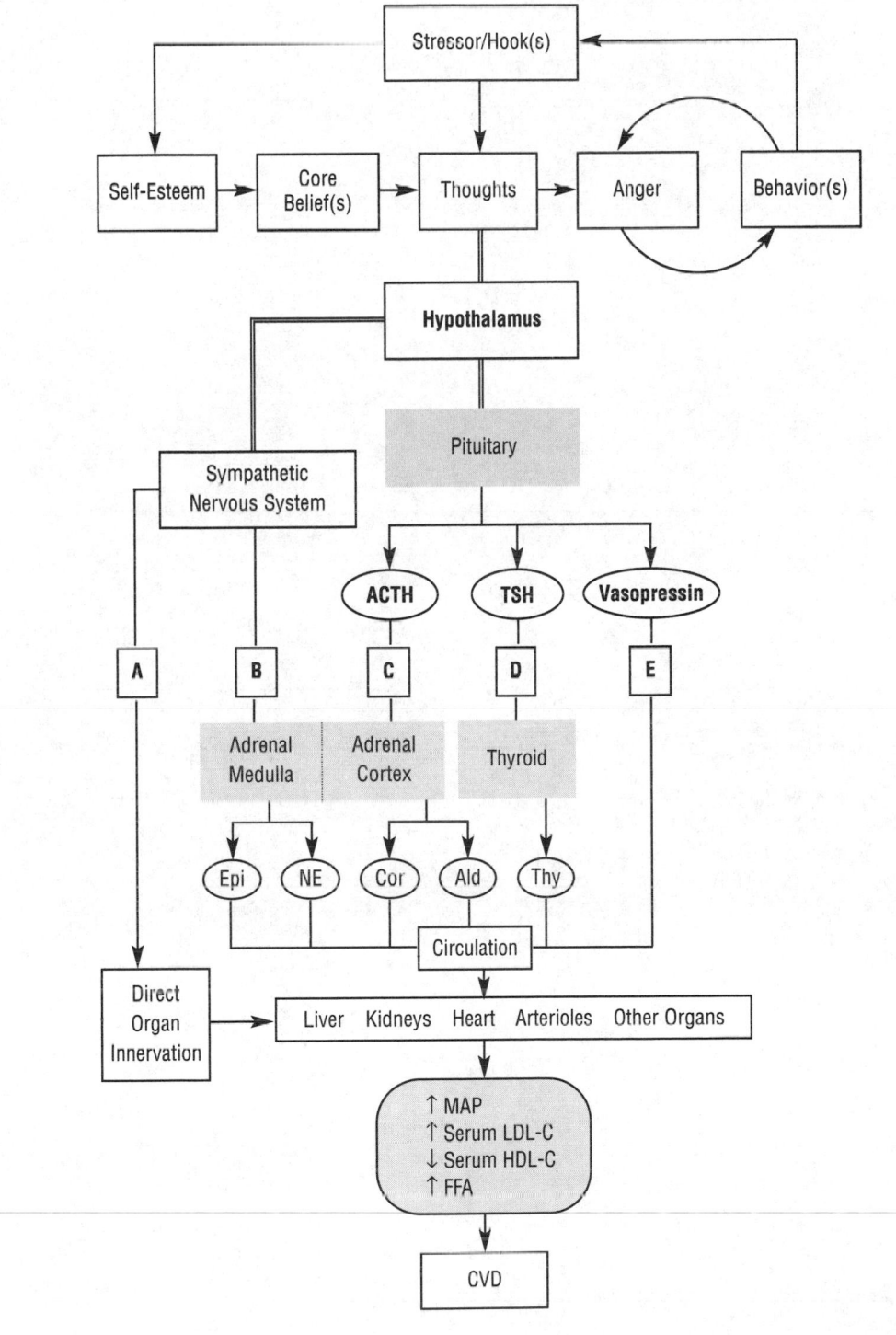

Appendix D

Coping with Terrorism and Other Traumatic Events

IN THE WAKE of September 11, 2001, the need for information and mental health skills that help people cope with catastrophic events became greater than ever. It is our hope that the following information will be useful.

What psychological reactions are we likely to experience following acts of terrorism?

We should expect to experience a full spectrum of strong emotions, ranging from stunned disbelief and shock to anger, grief, fear, numbness, guilt, and/or resolve. These feelings are normal. Some might experience post-traumatic stress disorder (PTSD), an understandable response to overwhelmingly dangerous and sudden events. Although PTSD is more likely to occur following stressful events, it is not inevitable.

Is the current state of mental health care in America adequate to the challenge of treating terrorism-related psychological problems?

It is not. There are presently too few mental health professionals to treat even the everyday mental disorders that are prevalent in the nation. Our best hope is to prevent mental illness by developing psychological and spiritual resilience and coping skills.

What we can do to help ourselves, our families, and our communities to cope?

1. *Accept the full range of feelings as normal.* At some point, when it is appropriate, allow yourself to feel the painful feelings, to cry, to shake, or to experience whatever naturally occurs. As calmly as possible, process what has happened by writing or talking about the troubling events—what happened, and *what you are thinking and feeling.* This kind of journaling/talking has been found to significantly improve mood and physical health, following an initial drop in mood as we confront the reality of what has happened. Feelings are part of who we are. Confronting the depths of painful feelings also enables us to discover our reserves of strength and to heal. Those who avoid painful feelings are paradoxically at higher risk for post-traumatic stress disorder. Be a resource for family and friends. Compassionately encourage others to communicate their feelings. Listen to and validate those feelings. It is gaining comfort with the full range of emotions that builds psychological resilience, not denying feelings.

2. *Keep what happened in perspective.* Terrorism is the work of evil that does not represent the majority of people in the world. Acts of terror are not personal, but reflect the pain and irresponsible scapegoating of the perpetrators. Despite the horror, most of the country is intact. We are a resilient nation and we will survive what has happened with resolve. What we stand for—decency and freedom—is stronger than fanaticism. Especially, hold an image of love and decency that is greater than the image of evil. This wholesome image might be of a loving God or of loving and decent people. Some find solace in the spiritual perspective that no eternal defeat befalls decent individuals.

3. *Keep a calm resolve, focusing on what you individually want to do,* be it giving blood or other donations, caring for loved ones,

consoling the bereaved, seeking justice, rededicating to the common good, praying for our leaders, etc.

4. *Guard your physical health*, especially as distress becomes prolonged. Exercise regularly, which expends the energy of stress. A brisk walk of twenty minutes or more on most days is remarkably therapeutic. This is especially important as we sit around the television watching distressing scenes. Stress that is not discharged physically becomes locked in the mind and body and may emerge later in the forms of nightmares, intrusive thoughts, anxiety, etc. Get adequate sleep and nourishment, avoiding as much as is prudent medications or substances that interfere with mental clarity and with the processing of the traumatic events.

5. *Avoid thoughts that excessively arouse the nervous system.* Such thoughts include *catastrophizing* ("This is awful. I can't stand it. I'm losing my mind."), *shoulds* ("I shouldn't be feeling so afraid or weak"), and *all-or-nothing* ("I'm either strong or I'm a weakling").

6. *Watch for subtle alterations in breathing.* Breathe abdominally, or slowly and quietly without moving the upper body. Remember to think of the area around your navel as if it were a balloon, inflating on the in-breath and deflating on the out-breath. This is important in helping to prevent panic attacks and many symptoms of anxiety. Following exposure to traumatic events, many people first alter the way they breathe, then experience panic attacks, then suffer dissociation and post-traumatic stress disorder. Other tips for coping with panic include: (a) Greet fear cordially. Say, "Hello, fear." Let it enter, flow with it like a reed blowing in the wind, knowing that even the worst panic attacks are simply stress responses that typically run their course in a few minutes. (b) Think, "This traumatic event is really happening. It is difficult, but I'll focus on what I need to do. I'll get through this." (c) Ground yourself, perhaps by touching a wedding band, rubbing your leg, saying a calming prayer, etc.

7. *Stengthen your faith*, through worship, prayer, family evenings at home, or any other method that reminds us there is a

larger order than the present crisis. Recommit to holy living. Create an inner peace of conscience that is steadfast in the face of chaos.

8. *When the crisis has passed, grieve.* Many who are so preoccupied with survival forget that something is always lost in trauma, something that requires grieving. Rituals and symbols of love, farewells, hope, and resolve often help.

9. *Do not allow yourself to be consumed with hatred.* It not only lowers us to the level of the perpetrators but also increases the risk of psychological illnesses such as post-traumatic stress disorder. We can resist terrorism and take strong countermeasures without hatred.

10. *Anticipate future occurrences of terrorism.* Be prepared, but do not obsess about their possibilities. Preparation might include storing, without hysteria, supplies of food, water, fuel, clothes, etc., to sustain one's family in the event of future upheavals. Once prepared, remind yourself and your family that wholesome recreation is not only permissible but is essential to maintain balance.

11. *Cultivate the attributes of resilient copers,* namely, reasoned optimism, self-esteem, flexibility, meaning and purpose, altruism, sense of beauty, morality, spirituality, sense of humor, sociability, emotional intelligence, calmness under duress, balanced living, and active problem solving (i.e., anticipating and actively planning for difficult times). Conversely, minimize isolation, severe emotions (e.g., excessive panic, guilt, or hatred), and avoidance/dissociation.

12. *Show physical and verbal affection to your family members to provide a sense of security.* Children should not be repeatedly exposed to media images of terrorism. Discuss what has happened after watching such scenes together once. Assure your children that very capable people are doing all they can to bring the perpetrators to justice and to protect us. Ask them what they think they can do to help themselves and their friends, family, and nation. Remember, active problem solving protects against psychological distress. Passivity and avoidance are risk factors.

13. *If symptoms do not resolve in a few weeks, become over-whelming, or interfere with your ability to work or relate to people, seek help from a mental health professional who specializes in treating post-traumatic stress disorder.* A range of new approaches can be very helpful. Bear in mind that a present trauma might reactivate unresolved past traumas. This can be a useful signal to resolve such emotional wounds. Signs of post-traumatic stress disorder include:

- Reexperiencing the distressing event(s) by intrusive thoughts, nightmares, flashbacks, etc.
- Arousal, including sleep difficulties, excessive anxiety, hypervigilance, increased startle response, or inability to concentrate
- Avoidance of any thing/person/activity that reminds us of the traumatic event, social withdrawal, emotional numbness, or a pessimistic inability to think of or plan for a normal future

What can we learn from resilient World War II survivors?

From interviewing WWII survivors who lived well-adjusted lives in the decades after combat, we have learned that there are certain recurring qualities that contribute to resiliency. The survivors did their duty without animosity and were men of faith, decency, and moral character. They maintained their sense of humor and hope. And they acknowledged their fears and then acted anyway.

Notes

Introduction

1. Research has linked excessive anger and hostility to death from all leading causes, not just heart disease.

Chapter 1: About Anger

1. S. Fried and P. Fried, *Bullies and Victims: Helping Your Child Survive the Schoolyard Battlefield* (New York: M. Evans, 1996).

2. For an overview of these personality disorders, see the Glossary or G. R. Schiraldi, *The Post-Traumatic Stress Disorder Sourcebook* (Los Angeles: Lowell House, 2000).

3. It is estimated that 10 percent of people in the United States have some form of neurological problem that impairs functioning. This rate is higher in prisons, nursing homes, rehabilitation centers, and shelters. A neuropsychologist and neuroimaging techniques are valuable resources.

4. For suggesting this approach, we're grateful to T. W. McKnight and R. H. Phillips, *How to Win the Love You Want* (New York: Galahad, 1998).

5. Cited in Dalai Lama, *The Art of Happiness* (New York: Riverhead, 1998), 123–24.

6. For an impressive review, see H. Kassinove, ed., *Anger Disorders: Definition, Diagnosis, and Treatment* (New York: Taylor and Francis, 1995). Cognitive-behavioral skills produce large effect sizes.

7. J. J. Gill et al., "Reduction in Type A Behavior in Healthy Middle Aged American Military Officers," *American Heart Journal* 110 (September 1985): 503–14.

8. S. E. Goodwin and M. J. Mahoney, "Modification of Aggression Through Modeling: An Experimental Probe," *Journal of Behavior, Therapy, and Experimental Psychiatry* 6 (1975): 200–202.

9. M. A. Schaeffer et al., "Effects of Occupational Based Behavioral Counseling and Exercise Interventions on Type A Components and Cardiovascular Reactivity," *Journal of Cardiopulmonary Rehabilitation* 8 (1988): 371–77.

10. For example, see M. Friedman et al., "Alteration of Type A Behavior and Its Effect on Cardiac Recurrences in Post Myocardial Infarction Patients: Summary Results of the Recurrent Coronary Prevention Project," *American Heart Journal* 112, no. 4 (1986): 653–65. Also see J. A. Blumenthal et al., "Stress Management and Exercise Training in Cardiac Patients with Myocardial Ischemia: Effects on Prognosis and Evaluation of Mechanisms," *Archives of Internal Medicine* 157, no. 19 (October 27, 1997): 2213–23. The former showed that Type A behavior could be reduced, and so doing significantly reduced the risk of a second heart attack. The latter study showed that stress management (relaxation, reducing hostility and depression) was more effective in reducing second heart attacks than even exercise or medication.

11. *Journal of Social Psychology*, 1933 (4): 285–309, p. 217.

Chapter 2: The Principles of Anger Management

1. Dalai Lama, *Healing Anger: The Power of Patience from a Buddhist Perspective* (Ithaca, NY: Snow Lion, 1997).

2. J. M. Schofield, "Address to the Corps of Cadets, August 11, 1879," *Bugle Notes* 90 (West Point, NY: U.S. Military Academy, 1998): 258.

3. F. C. Pogue, "George C. Marshall Global Commander," *The Harmon Memorial Lectures in Military History*, no. 10 (CO: United States Air Force Academy, 1968), 16; cited in "Center for Army Leadership," *Leadership* (Ft. Leavenworth, KS: U.S. Army Command and General Staff College), 93.

Chapter 3: Cooling Down

1. Edmund Jacobson, *You Must Relax*, 5th ed. (New York: McGraw-Hill, 1978).

Chapter 4: Calm Thinking

1. Adapted with permission from A. Ellis and R. Harper, *A New Guide to Rational Living* (North Hollywood, CA: Wilshire Book, 1975). Copyright by Albert Ellis Institute. Dr. Ellis also originated the *should* and *catastrophizing* distortions, rational emotive imagery, and rational role reversal, all adapted with permission from the same source.

2. Automatic thoughts and distortions are described in A. T. Beck, *Cognitive Therapy and the Emotional Disorders* (New York: Meridian, 1976). Dr. Beck originated most of the distortions commonly used today in cognitive therapy. The list of distortions and their definitions are adapted with permission from Dr. Aaron T. Beck, M.D. In this book, Dr. Beck first described personalization (personalizing) and polarized thinking (all-or-nothing). In A. T.

Beck, *Depression: Causes and Treatment* (Philadelphia: University of Pennsylvania Press, 1970), Dr. Beck originated selective abstraction (irritation fixation), arbitrary inference (jumping to conclusions or assuming), overgeneralization (overgeneralizing), magnification and minimization (similar to unfavorable comparisons), and inexact labeling (abusive labeling). As previously mentioned, Dr. Albert Ellis originated catastrophizing and shoulds (A. Ellis and R. Harper, *A New Guide to Rational Living*). Distortions were popularized in books such as M. McKay, M. Davis, and P. Fanning, *Thoughts & Feelings* (Oakland, CA: New Harbinger, 1981), which added blaming to the list of distortions, and D. Burns, *Feeling Good* (New York: New American Library, 1980), which added emotional reasoning (feelings passing as facts), mind reading, and fortune telling.

3. I've also liked the term *tunnel vision* to describe this distortion. A former student, who had been a sharpshooter and commando in the Iranian army, related: "Anger causes me to get tunnel vision. I do not see anything except destroying my opponent. It's like looking down the barrel of a gun and only seeing my enemy. Many times I have traveled this vicious tunnel as nice and very precious people pass by me, but I don't even see them or hear their comments. After my cruel mission is finished, I sit and feel ashamed that I totally ignored these people who were valuable and dear to me. Worse, sometimes I even hurt them although they did nothing wrong."

4. Albert Ellis and certain pastoral counselors have engaged in a warm debate over the years. Ellis asserts that no shoulds are reasonable, while the pastoral counselors disagree. It is difficult to argue that divine injunctions, such as one should not murder or cheat on a spouse, are not in humans' best interest. Even here, however, it is good to remind ourselves that some people, for their own reasons or lack of development, will not follow such injunctions. It has also been argued that people who develop to the point of saying, "I *want to* obey and *choose to* obey," are more positively motivated by desire, whereas people who obey because they *should* are more likely to be motivated by guilt. Finally, if divine injunctions are

beneficial, does that mean that all the shoulds that humans inflict upon others are?

5. Dr. Aaron T. Beck originated the idea of recording and evaluating thoughts. Various versions of the Daily Thought Record are found in: A. T. Beck et al., *Cognitive Therapy of Depression* (New York: Guilford, 1979); J. Scott, et al., eds., *Cognitive Therapy in Clinical Practice: An Illustrative Casebook* (New York: Routledge, 1989); A. T. Beck et al., *Cognitive Therapy of Substance Abuse* (New York: Guilford, 1993); J. S. Beck, *Cognitive Therapy: Basics and Beyond* (New York: Guilford, 1995); A. T. Beck and G. Emery, with R. L. Greenberg, *Anxiety Disorders and Phobias: A Cognitive Perspective* (New York: Basic, 1985); G. Emery, *Controlling Depression Through Cognitive Therapy: Clinician's Manual* (New York: BMA Audio Cassettes, Division of Guilford, 1982); W. Dryden and A. Ellis, "Rational-Emotive Therapy," in *Handbook of Cognitive-Behavioral Therapies*, ed. K. S. Dobson, ed. (New York: Guilford, 1988); and P. M. Lewinsohn et al., *Control Your Depression* (New York: Prentice Hall, 1986).

6. Dr. Aaron Beck originated the process of questioning to uncover core beliefs. See, for example, A. T. Beck et al., *Cognitive Therapy of Substance Abuse*. Also see J. S. Beck, *Cognitive Therapy: Basics and Beyond*, and D. Burns, *Feeling Good*.

Chapter 5: Self-Esteem

1. Recent research has shown that aggressive children are more likely to report feeling miserable, depressed, left out, and negative toward themselves.

2. This concept is rooted in Judeo-Christian theology, which holds that individuals are created in the image and likeness of God.

3. J. Gauthier, D. Pellerin, and P. Renaud, "The Enhancement of Self-Esteem: A Comparison of Two Cognitive Strategies," *Cognitive Therapy and Research* 7, no. 5 (1983): 389–98.

Chapter 6: Meditation

1. H. Benson, *Beyond the Relaxation Response* (New York: Berkley, 1984).

2. The teachings on Tibetan meditation incorporated into this chapter are adapted from Sogyal Rinpoche, *The Tibetan Book of Living and Dying* (New York: HarperCollins, 1993).

3. Ibid., 62.

4. Seeing clearly from such a vantage point permits one to recognize one's own insecurities and unrealistically high expectations. It also allows one to see the pain in an offender.

5. I have found this tai chi–like exercise to be a very good physical preparation for meditation. It is adapted from N. L. Tubesing and D. A. Tubesing, eds., "Clouds to Sunshine" exercise, *Structured Exercises in Stress Management*, vol. 3 (Duluth, MN: Whole Person Associates, 1994).

Chapter 7: Variations on Meditation

1. S. McNeal and C. Frederick, "Internal Self-Soothing: Other Implications of 'Inner Strength' with Ego States." Paper presented at the annual conference of the American Society of Clinical Hypnosis, Philadelphia, March 1994. Reprinted in M. Phillips and C. Frederick, *Healing the Divided Self: Clinical and Ericksonian Hypnotherapy for Post-Traumatic and Dissociative Conditions* (New York: Norton, 1995).

Chapter 8: Hot Buttons: Healing Hidden Wounds from the Past

1. J. Bradshaw, *Homecoming: Reclaiming and Championing Your Inner Child* (New York: Bantam, 1990).

2. "Second Annual Mental Health Awards," *Psychology Today* 34, no. 3 (May/June 2001): 46–51. Rogers was honored along with Dr. Albert Ellis and six others.

3. F. Rogers, *You Are Special: Words of Wisdom from America's Most Beloved Neighbor* (New York: Viking Penguin, 1994), 115.

4. Ibid., 123.

5. In our experience, the death of a child is one of the most difficult forms of loss. It is not unusual in such instances to feel angry with God for allowing this to happen and distant from God until this is resolved. I am reminded of an incident that I first reported in *Conquer Anxiety, Worry and Nervous Fatigue*. I asked my graduate class if anyone wished to demonstrate how cognitive restructuring is used in modifying anger. One student volunteered, and chose as the stressor the death of her brother, who fell to his death from a building. Her anger centered on his careless supervisors, her brother for not being careful, and God for letting the accident happen. It was the latter she chose to work with. Among her self-talk was the idea, "How could a loving God allow such a good twenty-nine-year-old man to die as he did?" As we pondered these thoughts, the idea came to my mind, which I shared, knowing her religious orientation: "How could a loving God allow a *perfect* thirty-three-year-old man to die as *He* did?" She reported later that that idea helped her dispel her anger in a profound and peaceful way for the first time in the year since her brother's death.

6. Bradley P. Barris, Ph.D., personal communication, July 2, 2001.

7. This section summarizes the work of Dr. James W. Pennebaker, *Opening Up: The Healing Power of Expressing Emotion* (New York: Guilford, 1997). Instructions for confiding in writing and the summary of supporting research are adapted with permission.

Chapter 9: Maintaining Equilibrium

1. In fact, exercise is the only known strategy to increase deep sleep in the elderly.

2. The "Pleasant Events Schedule" and the instructions for using it are adapted with permission from P. Lewinsohn et al., *Control Your Depression* (New York: Prentice Hall, 1986). © 1986 by Peter M. Lewinsohn.

Chapter 10: Peace Within

1. N. Cousins, *Human Options* (Toronto: George J. McLeod Limited, 1981), 45.

2. Dalai Lama, *A Policy of Kindness* (Ithaca, NY: Snow Lion, 1990), 104.

3. A. Petrie and J. Petrie, *Mother Teresa*, videocassette (San Francisco: Dorason Corporation, 1986).

4. Rogers, *You Are Special*, 163.

5. Ibid., 31.

6. O. Chambers, *My Utmost for His Highest* (Uhrichsville, OH: Barbour, 1963), 106. The next quotation is from page 134.

Chapter 11: Reducing Hostility

1. J. P. Sartre, *Anti Semite and Jew* (New York: Schocken Books, 1948), 13.

2. A. T. Beck, *Prisoners of Hate* (New York: HarperCollins, 1999), 184.

3. I. G. Opdyke, with J. Armstrong, *In My Hands: Memories of a Holocaust Rescuer* (New York: Anchor, 2001).

4. A. Schweitzer, *Reverence for Life* (New York: Hallmark Publishing, 1971), 31.

5. M. Silver, "Together Forever," *Sports Illustrated*, July 24, 2000, 93(4), 56–59.

6. C. Felton, "Finders Keepers?" *Readers Digest*, April 2001, 103–107.

7. P. Gulley, *Front Porch Tales* (Sisters, OR: Multnomah, 1997), 132.

8. This true story was written by aikido sensei Terry Dobson looking back at himself years prior. Adapted and reprinted

with permission from personal material from the estate of Terry Dobson.

9. Mother Teresa reminded us that if she hadn't helped the first dying person in Calcutta, she would have never helped the forty-two thousand. The habit of helping starts in simple ways, by the way we look at people, touch them, and speak to them.

10. Adapted Beck, *Prisoners of Hate*, 245.

11. The Judeo-Christian injunction to love one's enemies has much to speak for it. Not only does this approach prevent escalation of anger and permit the offender room to modify his behavior without defensiveness, but it also keeps us from sinking into hostility and thus becoming as troubled as the offender. One religion teacher became quite concerned about a student's hatred toward another girl who had stolen her boyfriend. When all else failed, he had her throw darts at a picture of the girl that was tacked to the wall. When this exercise seemed to provide the girl some satisfaction, the teacher removed the picture from the wall. Behind the picture was a picture of Jesus, with the inscription: "Inasmuch as you do it to the least of these, you do it unto me." As Hugh Nibley wrote, "We can afford the luxury of trusting our fellow-man only because we trust in God, who has assured us that if others let us down, he will make it up to us." (*Of All Things*, 2d ed. Salt Lake City, UT: Deseret Books, 1993, 23.)

12. I am reminded of the late Susie Graves, a dear friend. When shopping with her once, I noticed that everyone was smiling at her as we rode the escalator. I looked at her and saw that she had a sincere smile for each person passing in the opposite direction. Many Type As resist this drill at first, suspecting that others will ridicule them. They are usually pleasantly surprised to find that most people smile back at them.

13. Rogers, *You Are Special*, 104.

Chapter 12: Forgiving

1. If the offender can't listen, understand, or respond reasonably, you might want to bypass the first two bullets.

Chapter 13: Interpersonal Skills

1. The majority of spouse batterers desperately want to be loved and understood, but lack the skills to meet these goals. Fearing abandonment, they often try to dominate and control the other spouse, and erupt violently when their sense of control or acceptance is threatened.

2. Some of the leading researchers include J. Gottman, University of Washington; T. Huston, University of Texas at Austin; and H. Markman, S. Stanley, and S. L. Blumberg, University of Denver.

3. As a rule, men take longer to process emotional material, perhaps because the brains of men and women develop differently. Thus, it is wise to try to keep conflict as emotionally low key as possible, allowing men more time to process difficult issues.

4. Adapted with permission from Dr. E. James Lieberman. From E. J. Lieberman and K. Lieberman Troccoli, *Like It Is: A Teen Sex Guide* (Jefferson, NC: McFarland, 1998).

5. H. J. Markman, S. M. Stanley, and S. L. Blumberg, *Fighting for Your Marriage: Positive Steps for Preventing Divorce and Preserving a Lasting Love* (San Francisco: Jossey-Bass, 1994), 245.

6. Beck, *Prisoners of Hate*, 267.

7. W. P. Droubay, "Heart to Heart," *Ensign* (June 1997): 56–59.

8. M. Eastman with S. C. Rozen, *Taming the Dragon in Your Child: Solutions for Breaking the Cycle of Family Anger* (New York: Wiley, 1994). The form following these guidelines is patterned after Dr. Eastman's.

9. This approach is suggested by G. I. Latham, *The Power of Positive Parenting: A Wonderful Way to Raise Children* (North Logan, UT: P&T Ink, 1994).

10. You might encourage the children to establish their own system of rewards and consequences (e.g., ask them what nice things they might do for each other if they stick to the plan for a certain amount of time).

Chapter 14: Innovative Approaches

1. S. Stosny, *Treatment Manual of the Compassion Workshop* (Gaithersburg, MD: Compassion Power, 1995).

2. If you can't connect to a core value image, you might try eye movements. Think about what you are feeling (e.g., powerless or unlovable). Then think about what you would like to connect with (e.g., an image of feeling powerful or lovable). Experience all the negative thoughts, feelings, and physical sensations. While holding all of this in your mind, move two fingers back and forth across your visual field about twelve times, about 14 inches away from your eyes. Follow the movements with your eyes, holding your head still. Then let everything in your mind go ("blank it out") and notice what you get. The original negative image might have shifted; your mind may even have identified the image you are seeking. You can clear everything from your mind and repeat the eye movements until the desired image is obtained. The theory is that eye movements unlock frozen positive images in the mind and allow them to connect with present awareness.

3. P. Huggins, *Helping Kids Handle Anger* (Longmont, CO: Sopris West, 1998).

4. Imagery is very personal. If the turtle image does not appeal to you, you might prefer an image in nature, such as a cool lake.

5. The first five examples are adapted and reprinted with permission from M. H. Messer, *Soft Answers . . . They Turn Away Wrath* (Chicago: The Anger Institute, 2000). Excellent anger resources may be ordered from The Anger Institute; see Appendix B. 111 N. Wabash, Suite 1702, Chicago, IL 60602 (Tel: 312-263-0035).

6. These responses are suggested by Huggins in *Helping Kids Handle Anger*.

7. R. Kassinove, *Anger Disorders* (Washington, DC: Taylor & Francis, 1995), 168.

8. R. Rosenblatt, *Rules for Aging: Resist Normal Impulses, Live Longer, Attain Perfection* (New York: Harcourt, 2000), 3.

9. C. W. Hall, "The Noblest of Human Graces," *Readers Digest* (May 1975): 137–40.

10. Huggins, *Helping Kids Handle Anger*.

Chapter 15: Special Situations: Road Rage, Criticism, and Other Vexations

1. From Dr. Leon James and Dr. Diane Nahl, *Road Rage and Aggressive Driving* (Amherst, NY: Prometheus Books, 2000), 179. Copyright 2000. Reprinted by permission of the publisher.

2. Thanks to Denis Cerritos for suggesting this additional affirmation.

3. Huggins has suggested this reply in *Helping Kids Handle Anger*.

4. S. Horn, *Tongue Fu: How to Deflect, Disarm, and Defuse Any Verbal Conflict* (New York: St. Martin's Press, 1996). The first two examples are also from this source.

5. Fried and Fried, *Bullies and Victims*.

6. Huggins, *Helping Kids Handle Anger*.

Chapter 16: Caring for the Soul

1. J. B. Sprott and A. N. Doob, "Bad, Sad, and Rejected: The Lives of Aggressive Children," *Canadian Journal of Criminology* 42, no. 2 (2001): 123–33. Also see R. H. Durant et al., "Exposure to Violence and Victimization, Depression, Substance Use, and the Use of Violence by Young Adolescents," *Journal of Pediatrics* 137, no. 5 (November 2000): 707–13.

2. For a review, see D. B. Larson and S. S. Larson, *The Forgotten Factor in Physical and Mental Health: What Does the Research Show?* (Rockville, MD: National Institute for Healthcare

Research, 1994). D. B. Larson, a psychiatrist and former senior researcher for the National Institutes of Health, is currently president of the National Institute for Healthcare Research. Also see J. Gartner, D. B. Larson, and G. Allen, "Religious Commitment and Mental Health: A Review of the Empirical Literature," *Journal of Psychology and Theology* 19, no. 1 (1991): 6–25.

3. P. L. Benson and B. P. Spilka, "God-Image as a Function of Self-Esteem and Locus of Control," in *Current Perspectives in the Psychology of Religion,* H. N. Maloney, ed. (Grand Rapids, MI: Eerdmans, 1977), 209–24.

4. Although the concepts have been found in various cultures throughout history, Niebuhr is thought to have penned this prayer's first verse in 1926. The prayer is reprinted in R. A. Schuller, *Dump Your Hang-Ups without Dumping Them on Others* (Grand Rapids, MI: Flemming H. Revell, 1993), 198, with the following citation: *Big Book of AA* (New York: Alcoholics Anonymous World Service, Inc., 1966).

5. T. Moore, *Care of the Soul* (New York: HarperPerennial, 1992), 204, 214.

6. We have mentioned that sometimes people turn their backs on God for failing to protect them. "Bad things aren't supposed to happen to good people." "I could never reverence someone who lets suffering happen." These views assume that suffering does not have its purposes.

7. M. Muggeridge, "The Great Liberal Death Wish," *Imprimis* (Hillsdale College, Hillsdale, MI) (May 1979).

Chapter 17: Anticipating Angry Situations

1. D. Meichenbaum, *Stress Inoculation Training* (New York: Pergamon, 1985).

Glossary

Abuse Disrespectful and unkind treatment; intent to dominate, control, hurt, manipulate, or retaliate overshadows motive to know, enjoy, and appreciate someone. Types are:

- **Physical:** includes hitting, punching, slapping, choking, pushing, slamming, throwing, kicking, stomping, shaking, crushing, twisting limbs, burning, stabbing, cutting, shooting, pinching, mutilating; also includes throwing objects at someone

- **Emotional:** sometimes more subtle, includes belittling, criticism, talking down to someone, or name-calling; unfavorable comparisons to others; excessive expectations followed by contempt for imperfect performance; isolating (not permitting contact with friends or family, driving others away by gossip or lies); shouting; economic deprivation; neglect; ignoring feelings, needs, or reasonable requests; silent treatment; excessive teasing or disrespectful jokes; threats of any kind (e.g., to harm or leave); blaming the victim unreasonably for own or family's misfortunes; ridiculing something important to victim (values, beliefs, race, sexuality); punishing by withholding affection or appreciation; lying for the purpose of controlling;

humiliating another in public; trying to hurt someone by damaging their property or hurting their pets, children, etc.; interfering with another's privacy

- **Sexual:** rape, sadism, forced nudity, or committing other acts that are against a person's will

Accept To take in or receive gladly, approvingly; to believe in.

Aggression Forceful behavior. Aggression is considered a problem associated with anger when the intent is to deliberately hurt, destroy, bully, or dominate. Passive-aggressive behavior has the intent to control others, but in an indirect or confusing way (e.g., through sarcasm, teasing, silent treatment, etc.).

Anger An unpleasant and uncomfortable feeling arising from injury, mistreatment, opposition, etc. The word *anger* has the same root as anguish and angst.

Antisocial personality (sociopathy, psychopathy) A personality disorder where one rebels against social norms, deceives, is impulsive/reckless, is irritable and aggressive, disregards work/family obligations, and/or lacks conscience/remorse. Sociopaths can be cold, violent, hotheaded, indifferent to others' welfare, intimidating, and superficially charming. They seem dead to deep feelings (love, compassion, empathy, intimacy, remorse). They often appear confident, with an inflated sense of self; feel entitled to do or take what they want; and see compassion as a weakness. They are usually hostile, feeling that victims deserve what they get, that people need to be compelled to obey rules, and that aggression is needed for defense. Though apparently untroubled, it is not uncommon to find that they suffer from depression, anxiety, suicidal tendencies, and a borderline or narcissistic personality, which may explain their susceptibility to substance abuse. Their childhood was frequently chaotic or brutal, and rage might be a way to feel powerful. Brain damage, biological imbalances, and genetic vulnerabilities might also be risk factors.

Appreciate To rightly or favorably regard the quality of something; to enjoy.

Backstab To revile a person who is not present; backbite.

Bitterness Strong resentment, hostility, or hatred.

Borderline Personality A personality disorder marked by (1) poor self-esteem that might rise when a relationship is going well but fall with any threat of rejection; (2) a profound need for approval, coupled with a feeling of impending rejection; (3) a tendency to idealize lovers who are sufficiently devoted, but demonize and rage at the same lovers when they slight them; (4) self-destructive behavior in response to rejection or aloneness; and/or (5) feelings of emptiness, boredom, inability to be alone, and neediness. It is frequently seen in those whose homes were marked by abuse, abandonment, conflict, or neglect.

Bullying A form of abuse whereby the abuser aggressively attempts to harm and/or maintain power through size, age, strength, and/or gender; results in damaged self-esteem and withdrawal or aggression by victim, who is often vulnerable, isolated, and exposed (Fried and Fried).

Compassion Sorrow for the suffering of others and the deep desire to help.

Cynicism Disbelieving that people are good and sincere; assuming that people are selfish. In ancient Greek philosophy, Cynics held that virtue is the highest good and criticized people who were motivated by greed, material or selfish pleasures, etc.

Empathy Understanding and feeling for another's feelings or viewpoints.

Frustration The unpleasant feeling resulting when one is blocked from achieving an objective; can evolve into anger.

Grudge A feeling of ill will based upon a perceived wrong.

Hatred Loathing, strong dislike, ill will.

Hostility A generally stable, negative attitude of distrust and dislike toward people, plus the angry desire to punish.

Indignation "Righteous anger," seemingly arising from unjust, disrespectful, or ungrateful actions or treatment.

Malice Ill will, desire, and/or intention to do harm to another.

Misanthropy Dislike and distrust of people.

Narcissistic personality A personality disorder characterized by an air of superiority and the need for admiring attention, suggesting an underlying lack of self-love. Narcissists' self-absorption does not permit empathy or love for others. Instead, they will exploit others in order to succeed. Narcissism may be viewed as compensation for uncertain self-worth and as self-protection from vulnerability.*

Punish To cause someone pain or penalty for an offense, usually in a spirit of retribution ("make 'em pay") rather than correction. In contrast, discipline implies the intent to correct or improve behavior.

Rage Violent outbursts in which self-control is lost.

Resent Literally "to feel again"; this is the act of feeling and holding on to anger caused by a perceived hurt or offense; nursing a grudge like a festering sore.

Revenge The act of avenging or retaliating; of inflicting punishment, harm, or injury in return for an offense.

Revile To scold; to speak harshly or contemptuously to or about another person.

Sarcasm A cutting remark, with the intent to hurt.

Wrath Deep indignation expressed by the desire to punish or seek revenge.

---

*E. R. Parson, "Posttraumatic Narcissism: Healing Traumatic Alterations in the Self Through Curvilinear Group Psychotherapy," in *International Handbook of Traumatic Stress Syndromes,* eds. J. P. Wilson and B. Raphael (New York: Plenum, 1993), 821–40.

Bibliography

Beck, A. T. *Prisoners of Hate: The Cognitive Basis of Anger, Hostility, and Violence*. New York: HarperCollins, 1999.

Benson, H. *Beyond the Relaxation Response*. New York: Berkley, 1984.

Benson, P. L., and B. P. Spilka. "God-image as a Function of Self-esteem and Locus of Control." In *Current Perspectives in the Psychology of Religion*, edited by H. N. Maloney, 209–24. Grand Rapids, MI: Eerdmans, 1977.

Big Book of AA. New York: Alcoholics Anonymous World Service, Inc., 1966.

Blumenthal, J. A., et al. "Stress Management and Exercise Training in Cardiac Patients with Myocardial Ischemia: Effects on Prognosis and Evaluation of Mechanisms." *Archives of Internal Medicine* 157, no. 19 (October 27, 1997): 2213–23.

Borysenko, J. *Minding the Body, Mending the Mind*. New York: Bantam, 1987.

Bradshaw, J. *Homecoming: Reclaiming and Championing Your Inner Child*. New York: Bantam, 1990.

Chambers, O. *My Utmost for His Highest*. Uhrichsville, OH: Barbour, 1963.

Cousins, N. *Human Options*. Toronto: George J. McLeod Limited, 1981.

Dalai Lama. *A Policy of Kindness*. Ithaca, NY: Snow Lion, 1990.

————. *Healing Anger: The Power of Patience from a Buddhist Perspective*. Ithaca, NY: Snow Lion, 1997.

Deakin, D. "Couples: Seven Ways to Wreck Your Love Life." *The Washington Post*, 25 October 1983, Style Plus section.

Deffenbacher, J. L., et al. "Characteristics and Treatment of High-Anger Drivers." *Journal of Counseling Psychology* 47, no. 1 (2000): 5–17.

Droubay, W. P. "Heart to Heart." *Ensign* (June 1997): 56–59.

Durant, R. H., et al. "Exposure to Violence and Victimization, Depression, Substance Use, and the Use of Violence by Young Adolescents." *Journal of Pediatrics* 137, no. 5 (November 2000): 707–13.

Eastman, M., with S. C. Rozen. *Taming the Dragon in Your Child: Solutions for Breaking the Cycle of Family Anger*. New York: Wiley, 1994.

Felten, E. "Finders Keepers?" *Readers Digest* (April 2001), 103–7.

Frankl, V. *Man's Search for Meaning*. Boston: Beacon, 1959.

Fried, S., and P. Fried. *Bullies and Victims: Helping Your Child Survive the Schoolyard Battlefield*. New York: M. Evans, 1996.

Friedman, H., ed. *Hostility, Coping and Health*. Washington, DC: American Psychological Association, 1992.

Friedman, M., et al. "Alteration of Type A Behavior and its Effect on Cardiac Recurrences in Post Myocardial Infarction Patients: Summary Results of the Recurrent Coronary Prevention Project." *American Heart Journal* 112, no. 4 (1986): 653–65.

Gartner, J., D. B. Larson, and G. Allen. "Religious Commitment and Mental Health: A Review of the Empirical Literature." *Journal of Psychology and Theology* 19, no. 1 (1991): 6–25.

Gauthier, J., D. Pellerin, and P. Renaud. "The Enhancement of Self-Esteem: A Comparison of Two Cognitive Strategies." *Cognitive Therapy and Research* 7, no. 5 (1983): 389–98.

Gill, J. J., et al. "Reduction in Type A Behavior in Healthy Middle Aged American Military Officers." *American Heart Journal* 110 (September 1985): 503–14.

Goleman, G. *Emotional Intelligence.* New York: Bantam, 1995.

Goodwin, S. E., and M. J. Mahoney. "Modification of Aggression Through Modeling: An Experimental Probe." *Journal of Behavior, Therapy, and Experimental Psychiatry* 6 (1975): 200–202.

Gulley, P. *Front Porch Tales.* Sisters, OR: Multnomah, 1997.

Hall, C. W. "The Noblest of Human Graces." *Readers Digest* (May 1975): 137–40.

Horn, S. *Tongue Fu: How to Deflect, Disarm, and Defuse Any Verbal Conflict.* New York: St. Martin's Press, 1996.

Huggins, P. *Helping Kids Handle Anger: Teaching Self-Control.* Longmont, CO: Sopris West, 1998.

James, L., and D. Nahl. *Road Rage and Aggressive Driving: Steering Clear of Highway Warfare.* Amherst, NY: Prometheus Books, 2000.

Kassinove, H., ed. *Anger Disorders: Definition, Diagnosis, and Treatment.* Washington, DC: Taylor and Francis, 1995.

Larson, D. B., and S. S. Larson. *The Forgotten Factor in Physical and Mental Health: What Does the Research Show?* Rockville, MD: National Institute for Healthcare Research, 1994.

Larson, J., with C. Rodriguez. *Road Rage to Road-Wise.* New York: Tim Doherty, 1999.

Lewinsohn, P., et al. *Control Your Depression.* New York: Prentice Hall, 1986.

Lieberman, E. J., and K. Lieberman Troccoli. *Like It Is: A Teen Sex Guide.* Jefferson, N.C.: McFarland, 1998.

Markman, H., S. Stanley, and S. L. Blumberg. *Fighting for Your Marriage: Positive Steps for Preventing Divorce and Preserving a Lasting Love.* San Francisco: Jossey-Bass, 1994.

McNeal, S., and C. Frederick. "Internal Self-Soothing: Other Implications of 'Inner Strength' with Ego States." Paper presented at the annual society of the American Society of Clinical Hypnosis, Philadelphia, March 1994. Reprinted in M. Phillips and C. Frederick, *Healing the Divided Self: Clinical and Ericksonian Hypnotherapy for Post-Traumatic and Dissociative Conditions.* New York: Norton, 1995.

Messer, M. H. *Soft Answers . . . They Turn Away Wrath.* Chicago: The Anger Institute, 2000.

Moore, T. *Care of the Soul.* New York: HarperPerennial, 1992.

Muggeridge, M. "The Great Liberal Death Wish." *Imprimis* (Hillsdale College, Michigan) (May 1979).

Nibley, H. *Of All Things.* 2d ed. Salt Lake City, UT: Deseret Books, 1993.

Opdyke, I. G., with J. Armstrong. *In My Hands: Memories of a Holocaust Rescuer.* New York: Anchor, 2001.

Pennebaker, J. W. *Opening Up: The Healing Power of Expressing Emotion.* New York: Guilford, 1997.

Petrie, A., and J. Petrie. *Mother Teresa.* Videocassette. San Francisco: Dorason Corporation, 1986.

Rinpoche, S. *The Tibetan Book of Living and Dying*. New York: HarperCollins, 1993.

Rogers, F. *You Are Special: Words of Wisdom from America's Most Beloved Neighbor*. New York: Penguin, 1994.

Rosenblatt, R. *Rules for Aging: Resist Normal Impulses, Live Longer, Attain Perfection*. New York: Harcourt, 2000.

Sartre, Jean-Paul. *Anti Semite and Jew*. New York: Schocken Books, 1948.

Schaeffer, M. A., et al. "Effects of Occupational Based Behavioral Counseling and Exercise Interventions on Type A Components and Cardiovascular Reactivity." *Journal of Cardiopulmonary Rehabilitation* 8 (1988): 371–77.

Schiraldi, G. R. *Hope and Help for Depression: A Practical Guide*. Ellicott City, MD: Chevron, 1990.

———. *Facts to Relax By: A Guide to Relaxation and Stress Reduction*. Provo, UT: Utah Valley Regional Medical Center, 1996.

———. *Conquer Anxiety, Worry and Nervous Fatigue: A Guide to Greater Peace*. Ellicott City, MD: Chevron, 1997.

———. *The Post-Traumatic Stress Disorder Sourcebook: A Guide to Healing, Recovery and Growth*. Los Angeles: Lowell House, 2000.

———. *The Self-Esteem Workbook*. Oakland, CA: New Harbinger, 2001.

Schweitzer. A. *Reverence for Life*. New York: Hallmark Publishing, 1971.

Silver, M. "Together Forever," *Sports Illustrated* 93, no. 4 (24 July 2000): 56–59.

Sprott, J. B., and A. N. Doob. "Bad, Sad, and Rejected: The Lives of Aggressive Children." *Canadian Journal of Criminology* 42, no. 2 (2001): 123–33.

Stosny, S. *Treatment Manual of the Compassion Workshop*. Gaithersburg, MD: Compassion Power, 1995.

Vaillant, G. E. *Adaptation to Life*. Boston: Little, Brown and Co., 1977.

Webster's New World Dictionary of American English. New York: Prentice Hall, 1994.

Williams, R., and V. Williams. *Anger Kills: Seventeen Strategies for Controlling the Hostility That Can Harm Your Health*. New York: HarperCollins, 1993.

Wilson, J. P., and B. Raphael, eds. *International Handbook of Traumatic Stress Syndromes*. New York: Plenum, 1993.

About the Authors

Glenn R. Schiraldi, Ph.D., has served on the stress management faculties at the Pentagon, the International Critical Incident Stress Foundation, and the University of Maryland, where he received the Outstanding Teaching Award in the College of Health and Human Performance for teaching excellence. He is the author of numerous articles and books on human mental and physical health. His books on stress-related topics include *The Post-Traumatic Stress Disorder Sourcebook: A Guide to Healing, Recovery and Growth*; *Conquer Anxiety, Worry and Nervous Fatigue: A Guide to Greater Peace*; *Hope and Help for Depression: A Practical Guide*; *Facts to Relax By: A Guide to Relaxation and Stress Reduction*; and *The Self-Esteem Workbook*. His book-writing excellence has been recognized by various scholarly and popular sources, including *The Washington Post*, *American Journal of Health Promotion*, the *Mind/Body Health Review*, and the *International Stress and Tension Control Society Newsletter*.

Glenn is a graduate of the U.S. Military Academy, West Point, and holds graduate degrees from Brigham Young University (summa cum laude) and the University of Maryland. While serving at the Pentagon, he helped to design and implement a series of prototype courses in stress management for the Department of the Army—including hostility/anger management and communication skills.

Serving at the University of Maryland since 1980, he has pioneered a number of mind/body courses that have taught skills to a wide range of adults to prevent stress-related mental and physical illness. Because of his expertise in practical skill building to prevent mental illness, he was invited to join the Board of Directors, Depression and Related Affective Disorders Association, at Johns Hopkins University and presently serves in this position. He also serves on the editorial board of the *International Journal of Emergency Mental Health*.

Glenn has addressed clinicians, educators, and the lay public in a variety of forums, including radio, television, and national conventions.

His research interests at the University of Maryland center on personality and stress, including anger/hostility, resilience, post-traumatic stress, self-esteem, depression, and anxiety.

Melissa Hallmark Kerr, Ph.D., is an experienced and compassionate public and community health practitioner with a research focus on stress and mental health and a strong background in physiology and biology. Her passion is bridging the gap between academia and the needs of the community. She is the president of Kerr and Associates: Positive Youth Development Specialists, the mission of which is to build the capacity of youth-serving organizations to evaluate the effectiveness of programs using a practical evaluation model. She has taught a wide variety of college health courses at the University of Maryland and Anne Arundel Community College. She also has extensive health counseling experience in cardiac rehabilitation, nutrition, and exercise. One who practices what she preaches regarding mind/body health, she completed the Hawaii Ironman Triathlon in 1991 and is perpetually reading and learning. In addition to being an award-winning teacher, she is also a gifted scholar and writer.

Index